Praise for *Damnation Island*

"In her fine new book . . . Stacy Horn lucidly, and not without indignation, documents the island's bleak history, detailing the political and moral failures that sustained this hell, failures still evident today in the prison at Rikers Island."
—*The New York Times Book Review*

"*Damnation Island* should be your page-turning horror read for the summer. Horn's book is uniquely arranged almost like a guide book, venturing from one institution to the next, discovering intimate stories of mayhem and malfeasance more unbelievable than the last."
—*The Bowery Boys* podcast

"[A] fascinating look at a piece of nearly forgotten New York City history— one that will make you thankful for modern conveniences."
—*Mental Floss*, Best Books of 2018

"Horn creates a vivid and at times horrifying portrait of Blackwell's Island (today's Roosevelt Island) in New York City's East River during the late 19th century . . . with relevance for persistent debates over the treatment of the mentally ill and incarcerated."
—*Publishers Weekly*

"Stacy Horn's history of Blackwell's Island is a shocking tale, and an invaluable account that will reward anyone with an interest in the history of New York."
—Simon Baatz, *New York Times* bestselling author of *For the Thrill of It*

"This is an essential—and heartbreaking—book for readers seeking to better understand contemporary public policy." —*Booklist*, starred review

T0021507

"Horn brings this subject to light in stunning detail. Readers will instantly see how this history continues to haunt us, as the boundaries between the four classes of people on the island (the poor, the mad, the sick and the criminal) are, in the public imagination, as blurred as ever."

—*BookPage*

"Riveting. Horn brings alive this forgotten history and her extraordinary book has far-reaching significance not only for the past but for the future."

—Jan Jarboe Russell, *New York Times* bestselling author of *The Train to Crystal City*

"Teeter-tottering between a history textbook and a murder mystery, Stacy Horn's *Damnation Island* is fast moving and entrenched in detail . . . What's even more horrifying—it's all real . . . These days, the island is a residential community dotted with scenic parks and landmarks. But history buffs will be terrified by what occurred there a century ago."

—Brianne Kane, *BUST*

"Blackwell's Island's descent into darkness is chronicled with clarity and conscience by master storyteller Stacy Horn. No one who has taken that journey with her will return the same."

—Teresa Carpenter, Pulitzer Prize winner and editor of *New York Diaries: 1609 to 2009*

"A stunning examination of bureaucracy gone wrong, and the evolution of the place we now call Roosevelt Island."

—*Salon*

"At Blackwell's, the inmates really were running the asylum. An important piece of history in public medicine, *Damnation Island* weaves a compelling narrative with threads of thorough research and realism."

—Julie Holland, MD, author of *Weekends at Bellevue*

"Stacy Horn is the perfect Virgil for this chilling, vivid, and enthralling journey through the Inferno that was 19th-century Blackwell's Island."
　　　—Gary Krist, *New York Times* bestselling author of *Empire of Sin*

"Stacy Horn has given us the short tour of the Island. But what we learn is enthralling; it is well worth the trip."　　　—*New York Journal of Books*

"Horn engagingly explores a history that, perhaps surprisingly, extended into the 1960s."　　　—*Kirkus Reviews*

"Horn reveals how official assurances hid cruel indifference to the mentally ill. More than a diligent exposé, *Damnation Island* presents a cautionary tale for what could happen even now, informing and educating in a way that urges us toward humbling self-reflection."
　　　—Katherine Ramsland, professor of forensic psychology at DeSales University and author of *Confession of a Serial Killer*

"Revelatory. What occurred during the 19th and early 20th centuries in the prisons, hospitals, and insane asylum on the New York City spit of land that is now home to the fashionable Roosevelt Island constitutes the stuff of nightmares."
　　　—Steve Weinberg, author of
Taking on the Trust: The Epic Battle of Ida Tarbell and John D. Rockefeller

"A riveting character-driven dive into 19th-century New York and the extraordinary history of Blackwell's Island. Stacy Horn has an uncanny knack for making history come alive."
　　　—Laurie Gwen Shapiro, author of
The Stowaway: A Young Man's Extraordinary Adventure to Antarctica

"Blackwell's Island and its troubled history haunt New York City. Who better to delve into Damnation Island's many-layered secrets than one of America's foremost storytellers, Stacy Horn."

—Philip Dray, author of
At the Hands of Persons Unknown: The Lynching of Black America

"*Damnation Island* tells the real story of how America has treated its poor, its tired, and its huddled masses: with petty cruelty, often in the name of Christian charity. A gripping and compelling read."

—Mikita Brottman, author of *The Maximum Security Book Club*

"[Horn] meticulously reconstructs the long-since-demolished structures of Blackwell's Island—and gives a sense of the people both operating those institutions and trapped within them . . . The most discomfiting parts of New York City's history can also make for gripping, compelling drama."

—*Curbed New York*

DAMNATION ISLAND

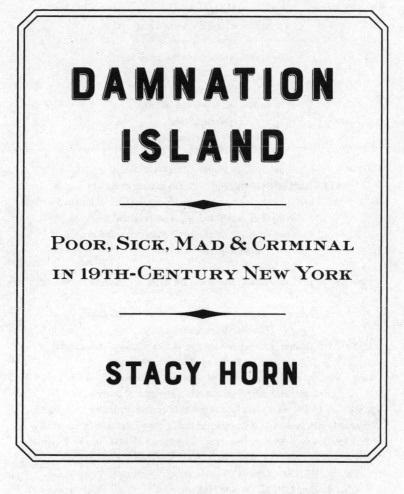

DAMNATION ISLAND

Poor, Sick, Mad & Criminal
in 19th-Century New York

STACY HORN

ALGONQUIN BOOKS
OF CHAPEL HILL
2019

Published by

ALGONQUIN BOOKS OF CHAPEL HILL
Post Office Box 2225
Chapel Hill, North Carolina 27515-2225

a division of
WORKMAN PUBLISHING
225 Varick Street
New York, New York 10014

First paperback edition, Algonquin Books of Chapel Hill, May 2019.
Originally published in hardcover by Algonquin Books of Chapel Hill in May 2018.
Printed in the United States of America.
Published simultaneously in Canada by Thomas Allen & Son Limited.
Design by Steve Godwin.

The Library of Congress has catalogued the hardcover edition as follows:

Library of Congress Cataloging-in-Publication Data
Names: Horn, Stacy, author.
Title: Damnation Island : poor, sick, mad & criminal in 19th-century
New York / by Stacy Horn.
Description: First edition. | Chapel Hill, North Carolina : Algonquin Books
of Chapel Hill, 2018. | Includes bibliographical references.
Identifiers: LCCN 2017052414 | ISBN 9781616205768 (hardcover : alk. paper)
Subjects: LCSH: French, William Glenney, 1814–1895. | Psychiatric hospitals—
New York (State)—New York—19th century—History. | Mental illness—Treatment—
New York (State)—New York—19th century—History. | Roosevelt Island
(New York, N.Y.)—19th century—History.
Classification: LCC RC445.N68 H67 2018 | DDC 362.2/1/097471—dc23
LC record available at https://lccn.loc.gov/2017052414

ISBN 978-1-61620-935-3 (PB)

10 9 8 7 6 5 4 3 2 1
First Paperback Edition

To all those who have ever
been judged unworthy.

CONTENTS

PROLOGUE

———————◆———————

WORKERS FOR THE Edison Electric Illuminating Company had spent more than a year ripping up the streets of lower Manhattan. The miles of cable that now lay unseen somewhere beneath their feet were making some people nervous. Two weeks before the new lamps were to be lit for the first time, the *New York Times* ran a story about horses that had been shocked on one of the blocks within the electrified grid. Absurd, Edison Electric responded. The conductors were buried two feet underneath the street, and encased in an iron pipe a quarter of an inch in diameter. Even if the pipe broke, the current would "scatter through the earth" rendering it utterly harmless. Anything could have spooked those horses.

The first test of electric light distributed via a central power station in New York City would go ahead as planned, on September 4, 1882.

On Monday afternoon at 3 p.m. the switch was thrown. Four-hundred lamps for eighty-five initial customers came to life, powered by six 27-ton, exuberantly named dynamos (today called generators). One of those customers was the *New York Times*. A grateful reporter wrote about working that night by light as "bright as day . . . without a particle of flicker, and with scarcely any heat to make the head ache." The new lights also lit up their rooms without the nauseating smell of the gaslights that electricity replaced. That December, a vice president of Edison's company wrapped his family's Christmas tree with eighty red, white, and blue light bulbs, and placed it on a revolving pine box. As the tree turned, the tiny lights went off and on, creating a "continuous twinkling of dancing colors" for his lucky children, and neighbors who strolled by for a peek inside. Everything, "all the lights and the fantastic tree itself with its starry fruit," which "kept going by the slight electric current brought from the main office on a filmy wire," so delighted a *Detroit Post and Tribune* reporter who was in New York that he could "hardly imagine anything prettier."

The city itself became a fantastic display as Edison and his competitors raced to illuminate all the streets. An editor visiting from London described the sight: "The effect of the light in the squares of the Empire City can scarcely be described, so weird and so beautiful is it." What some had feared, he saw as magical. "Enormous standards, rising far above the trees, are erected in the centre of each square. From these standards the light is thrown down upon the trees in such a way as to give them a fairy-like aspect . . . the shadows they cast on the pavement below appear very like living objects."

As time went on, more and more outdoor lamps lit up Manhattan, and by 1884 the "bright, white moonlight effect" could be seen for miles around, a glow that illuminated the city every evening, like a brilliant cloud.

That same year, the City of New York sent tens of thousands of people to Blackwell's Island, a narrow, two-mile-long strip in the East River where they'd built a "Lunatic Asylum," an "Almshouse for the Poor," two penal institutions, and over half a dozen hospitals for different classes of inmates. For those who caught an evening glimpse the night before being ferried across, it might have felt like they were being carried away from a radiant future that they would never inhabit. Instead, they were transported into the dank, nauseating, gas- and kerosene-lit past of Blackwell's Island, where they would be swallowed up—the enchanted, incandescent island of Manhattan in fact lost to many of them forever.

Those sent to the prisons, or even the Lunatic Asylum, could at least entertain a hope of one day getting out, assuming they weren't committed during a cholera outbreak which could kill them, or housed with a murderous inmate, who might do the same. But a great number of them, especially the unfortunates sent to the Almshouse, were generally too old or their bodies too broken to hope they would ever return to the bright city again. Their prospect for recovery had been judged so unlikely that someone had written *Future Doubtful*, or worse, *Permanently Dependent*, on their application for relief. For them, the Almshouse would be their last stop before death, dissection, and a burial in the potter's field.

Initial planners for Blackwell's would have been mortified at how wretched and deadly conditions there had become. When the island was bought by the city for $32,500 in 1828 (they would end up paying $20,000 more to settle a lawsuit), their goal was to relieve the crowded conditions at Manhattan's Bellevue, which in addition to being a hospital was also the location of the city's Penitentiary, the Lunatic Asylum, an Almshouse for the poor, and the Workhouse, a prison for people convicted of minor crimes. As the city had grown, so had the number of the poor, the lunatic, and the criminal, all of whom had to be treated somewhere when they got sick.

"Why have we not establishments worthy of our city?" an expert they would consult later asked, summing up just what legislators had been thinking at the time. Their idea was to move the sick, mad, and punishable away from the general population and into the more humane, stress-free, and healthful environment of this lush, pastoral island, thick with fruit trees, where they could be classified according to their affliction or crime, installed in their respective institutions, controlled, and finally reformed. The inmates would get all the benefits of modern science and a chance at a future, and except for the employees of the institutions, no one need be troubled about their existence ever again. The island also conveniently had stone quarries that could serve the dual purpose of providing the city with the materials for the buildings, and the prisoners and the poor with a useful occupation: breaking, blasting, and preparing rocks.

Everyone was in high spirits on that promising day when the cornerstone of the first institution was laid. John Stanford, the city's prison chaplain, thanked God for teaching America "how to season justice with mercy," and a confident Mayor William Paulding Jr. told the assembled crowd of guests that their state-of-the-art establishment would "prove an honor to our city." What could be more restorative for the unfortunates of the burgeoning metropolis, it was reasoned, than the peaceful, verdant island in the East River, tucked safely away from vice and crime between two swiftly running channels, surrounded by picturesque sailboats, ferries, and steamers, and the wooded reaches of upper Manhattan and Queens behind them?

Blackwell's Island was an extension of everything the New World offered, poured into 147 acres. Even the marginalized and maligned would have it better here and nothing less than the latest scientific methods would be employed to give them a chance to turn their lives around. On the Island everyone would be tended to in brand-new institutions with pioneering facilities. Whether they were consigned there for humane punishment, healing or relief, this was America, and here in America we were going to do everything better. The mayor and his fellow dignitaries crossed the river back to Manhattan satisfied that they'd put the largest city of the expanding young country firmly on the path of enlightened reform.

DAMNATION ISLAND

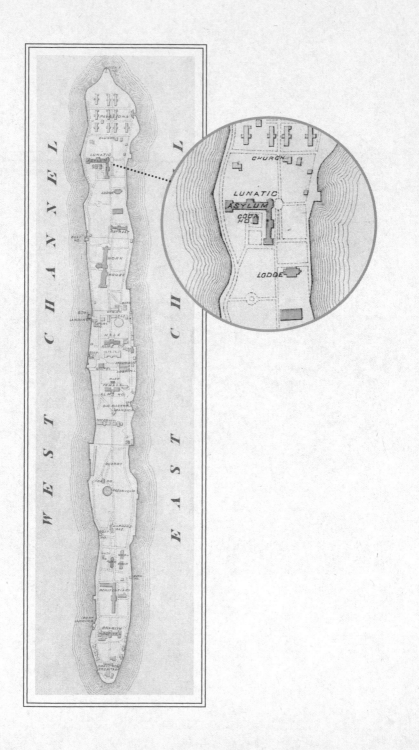

I

THE NEW YORK CITY LUNATIC ASYLUM

———◆———

OPENED ON BLACKWELL'S ISLAND 1839,
TO ACCOMMODATE NEW YORK CITY'S
LUNATIC POOR

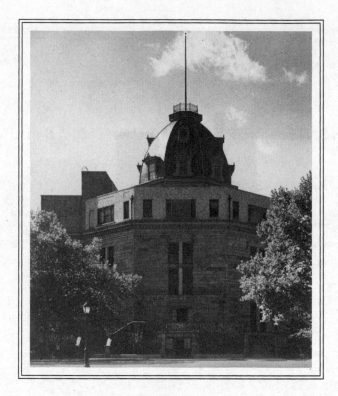

REVEREND WILLIAM GLENNEY FRENCH

The Blackwell's Island Episcopal Missionary from 1872 to 1895

HE WOULD CROSS and re-cross the East River thousands of times, including the day before his last on earth. It was a short journey, less than a quarter of a mile, and it wouldn't give him a lot of time to think. But on his first voyage, as he traveled to Blackwell's Island to begin what would become the most important mission of his life, the Reverend William Glenney French was likely full of the same sense of hope and aspiration that followed the mayor and his fellow officials back to New York City over forty years earlier.

In 1872 New York was exploding with realized potential, and the promise of unimaginable delights still to come, like the blazing electric lights that Edison would bring to light their race to the future. The Metropolitan Museum of Art had opened, immediately putting itself on the world-museum map by snatching a collection of priceless Cypriot antiquities out of the grasp of curators in France, Russia, and England. "The trustees of American museums are more enterprising," one paper fumed with envy. Businessmen on the Fulton Ferry could watch the daily progress on the Brooklyn Bridge, as laborers and stonemasons got to work on the towers, blasting through old docks, early shipwrecked vessels, anchors and chains. Over at 195 Broadway, Western Union, one of the companies that symbolized all that was thrilling about America, had commenced construction on what would become the first entrant in the architectural race to the skies, a new office building that would reach up ten stories and further by adding a clock tower.

Still, a mission on Blackwell's Island was a potentially lethal assignment. The first Jesuit missionary to go to Blackwell's died after contracting typhoid fever, followed by three more who would also die over the next three years. Anyone could fall. Dr. Moses Ranney, the resident physician of the Lunatic Asylum, and his assistant, Dr. A. Falls Marvin, both died of typhus in 1864. But French was tenacious, with a will as strong as the steel that would soon allow New York to fling itself up into the heavens and across the river as the city completed what was then the world's longest suspension bridge. He never backed down from a challenge.

A few years after his ordination, French was sent to a remote valley in rural North Carolina to establish a monastic community. To get from Manhattan to the sparsely populated region along the Watauga River, he boarded one steamship after another, then several trains, before walking roughly 196 miles alongside a two-horse wagon from Raleigh to the place they would call Valle Crucis. The next three punishing years were spent digging out and replacing brick from cellar walls, chopping wood, building walks, traveling miles through the mountains to visit his flock, with often only a biscuit and some mush to sustain him, and in a coat he'd made from a discarded blanket.

When the New York Protestant Episcopal City Mission Society offered French the position as a missionary on Blackwell's Island, he didn't hesitate. Two weeks later, and only days after celebrating his fifty-eighth birthday, Reverend French boarded the ferry at Twenty-Sixth Street, confident that he would not fail at what he was about to begin, just as certain as the mayor and the city planners had been when they first envisioned what they would build on Blackwell's Island.

THE NEW YORK City Lunatic Asylum looks so idyllic in early paintings and drawings, and that was exactly what the municipal authorities intended it to be. Before plans for the structure were submitted, a trip was made to an asylum in Philadelphia, now known as the Friends Hospital. Founded by Quakers in 1813, their asylum was based on what came to be known as "moral treatment," which had evolved from reforms begun in England and France, and elsewhere. It was the new scientific approach which New York City aimed to fully embrace.

Insanity was once believed to be due to a lack of faith, or demonic influence and possession, and it was treated by bleeding, starvation, prison cells, and straitjackets. Moral treatment was kinder and more humane, and therapy was focused on the patient's emotional and spiritual needs. There would be no more iron wristlets or leg-locks or bleedings; instead inmates would be cared for with exercise, self-esteem-building work, and amusements. "Never for a moment should it be forgotten, that insanity is a disease," was now the prevailing belief, and if we treat patients like fellow human beings they will respond with humanity.

Moral treatment also dictated the design of the buildings that would house the inmates, reflecting the city planners' faith in classification, institutionalization, and control. Their criteria were often conflicting, however. For instance, they wanted the Asylum to feel more home-like. It should be set in the country and restful, and "be as little like the Penitentiary as possible." There were to be no more than 250 patients, and each would get their own room with a window and access to a wash closet. But the plan also called for a grand and imposing structure, in order to make the inmates easier to control. A "great show of power," reflected in part by an awesome structure, they believed, would help "in subduing the violence of patients." That sounds a little stressful, and less humane.

Still, it was going to be better than prison, which is where the insane were often sent until 1827, when an "An Act concerning Lunatics" was passed, forbidding the mentally ill from being "confined in any prison, gaol or house of correction, or confined in the same room with any person charged with, or convicted of, any criminal offense."

Accordingly, design elements that had any suggestion of a prison were avoided. Small openings in the doors to the inmates' rooms would no longer be allowed. "To be looked at in this manner like a wild animal, is sufficient to excite the indignation of any one, and there is nothing more calculated to render the lunatic fierce and reckless or the attendant careless and cruel." Sash windows with iron instead of wood surrounding the windowpanes were used instead of bars.

There had also once been an accepted theory that the insane were not affected by variation of temperature, and so proper heating and ventilation had never been a high priority. "The error arose probably," wrote Dr. James Macdonald, an attending physician at the Bloomingdale Asylum who was advising New York's municipal authorities on the design, "from seeing one violent maniac, who generated an extraordinary degree of animal heat, bear and even seek the extremes of cold. Others suffer from cold who have not the intelligence to take cognizance of what causes them to suffer," and so would endure freezing temperatures "without uttering a complaint." This asylum would be properly heated in the winter, and have plenty of windows placed to provide for cross breezes in the summer.

A chapel was also part of the original plan. Most people practiced one form of religion or another, Macdonald reasoned, and "to deprive them of this privilege when removed from home and from the natural objects of their affection, will be to deprive them of one of the few consolations that should be left."

In the end, architect Alexander Jackson Davis was also influenced by the County Asylum at Hanwell in England. The original plan called for a series of wings forming the letter U, but it was eventually scaled back. At first only one wing was built, then two, which came together at right angles to each other, one for the men and one for the women. These two wings met at a fifty-foot-high octagon, which served as a central administration building with offices, storerooms, a sewing room, and the home of the resident physician who ran the Asylum. The crenellated patterns along the tops of the outer structures gave the Asylum a castle-like appearance, creating the imposing air advocated by some—although not Macdonald—who proposed a group of smaller, separate buildings. As planned, the Asylum was built entirely from thousands of tons of stone quarried on the island, a Precambrian rock called Fordham gneiss.

Although Dr. Macdonald reached for a note of realism when presenting his recommendations, it's clear he was confident the asylum on Blackwell's could become a beacon for all the world. "All plans for asylums yet offered or carried into effect, either in this or other countries, are not without defects. Nor do we flatter ourselves that our plan will be faultless, but it will be our endeavor so to profit by all preceding inquiries as to avoid errors and adopt improvements; and above all to adapt our building to its inmates."

But it all went south almost immediately. Only three years after the Lunatic Asylum opened in 1839, Charles Dickens visited and wrote that "everything had a lounging, listless, madhouse air . . . The moping idiot, cowering down with long disheveled hair; the gibbering maniac, with his hideous laugh and pointed finger; the vacant eye, the fierce wild face. . . . There they were all . . . in naked ugliness and horror."

The Asylum was doomed by two fatal flaws in the plan. First, the commissioners appointed to manage the institutions on Blackwell's drastically underestimated the need, a miscalculation they would make repeatedly as the island grew to accommodate an average of 7,000 people daily, across all the institutions. The commissioner positions were political appointments and the men weren't necessarily chosen for their expertise. But they hired everyone else who worked on the Island, and made most of the important operational decisions. The wardens, physicians, and superintendents who actually lived and worked on the Island had to appeal to them for all their needs. In the early years the commissioners reported to the Common Council, the legislative branch of New York at the time. Later, they reported to the mayor, who'd taken over making their appointments.

The initial asylum structure was built to accommodate 200 patients, which was within the parameters recommended by all the arbiters of moral treatment at that time. And while the Common Council and the commissioners knew they'd eventually have to provide for a larger population, they thought that would be enough for a while (it was also originally going to be twice the size, with two more wings). But no one really had an accurate sense of just what percentage of the population was, in

today's terms, suffering from mental disorders. In 1858 it was estimated
it to be .002 percent. Today around 28 percent of Americans suffer from
some form of anxiety disorder, an affliction that would have been enough
to get you committed in the nineteenth century. On the Asylum's very first
day of operation, June 10, 1839, they came right up against their maximum
when 197 patients—116 women and 81 men—were transferred from Bellevue to Blackwell's.

The commissioners immediately started adding additional structures.
A Mad House for the most violent and disturbed cases was quickly erected
and was so inadequate to the need that inmates were sleeping in the corridors, prompting one of the commissioners appointed to overseeing Blackwell's to call it a "disgrace to the institution." It was replaced in 1848 by a
seemingly more humane structure called the Lodge. Then the Retreat was
added, likely named after the York Retreat in England, which pioneered
moral treatment. The Retreat was built to house chronic cases, those who
were suicidal and generally too "noisy" and unhinged for the main Asylum, but not as violent as the people sent to the Lodge. After that, whenever
things got really bad they'd throw up smaller shelters they called pavilions. These were installed along the northern shore of the Island and were
nothing more than wooden shanties. While they were built to hold fifty of
what were designated "quieter" cases, they frequently housed seventy-five
to ninety or more.

The second great flaw was putting the Asylum under the management
of the same commissioners who ran the Penitentiary (and later the Workhouse and the Almshouse for the Poor) and then isolating these different
populations on the same small island. Although the insane were no longer
thrown in prison (mostly), the criminal and the insane still formed one
group in people's minds, along with the poor, who were often thought of
as defacto "guilty." The arrangement on Blackwell's Island only reinforced
this devastating association, which persists to this day. The mentally ill are
dangerous and poor people are thieves in disguise.

That tragic relationship was taken literally. To deal with their overcrowding issues, available space within the various institutions was often

used interchangeably. When needed, patients from the Lunatic Asylum (including those who were deemed incurable) were moved to the Alms-house or into garrets in the Workhouse; Almshouse inmates were relo-cated to the Workhouse, and Charity Hospital patients who couldn't be made whole again might end up anywhere except the Penitentiary.

The worst decision to ever come out of this disastrous alliance was to put convicts to work in the Lunatic Asylum as nurses and attendants. It would save the city money, the commissioners reasoned, and as long as they were careful, what could possibly go wrong?

The men actually running the Asylum knew better. One early resident physician, Moses Ranney, pointed out what should have been terribly obvi-ous: "That the same individuals who were committed in the City as crimi-nals, and required an armed keeper in the Penitentiary, were sent here to take charge of a class who require the most mild and soothing treatment." He was ignored.

Ranney didn't give up. Year after year he begged the commissioners to reconsider. He told them how the convicts stole clothes from the patients, and anything else they could get their hands on. One night a particularly vulnerable patient who'd just been admitted found herself cornered in a room with a worker from the Penitentiary who held her down and com-pletely shaved her head. The convict planned to sell her ringlets to a wig maker. "The idea that the citizens of New York could not afford, or were unwilling to have suitable attendants for the insane," Ranney argued, "is ridiculous in the extreme." In reality, the cost for the care of the insane was down to 18 cents a day ($4.88 in today's dollars) and the commission-ers were quite proud of that accomplishment, even though it was already clear that this amount wasn't close enough to even feed everyone properly.

In 1848 Ranney took such an audacious step that it's surprising it didn't cost him his job. He invited Thomas Story Kirkbride to tour the Asylum. Kirkbride was the superintendent of the Pennsylvania Hospital for the In-sane, a founder of the Association of Medical Superintendents of American Institutions for the Insane (AMSAII), and the preeminent authority and proponent of moral treatment in the United States.

Ranney knew full well what Kirkbride would see. It can only be assumed that what happened next was precisely what Ranney had intended. Perhaps he and Kirkbride planned it together. On May 8, at a meeting of the AMSAII and in front of most of the superintendents of all the asylums in the United States, including Moses Ranney, Kirkbride stood and related the deplorable state of affairs at the Asylum in New York City. Ranney couldn't have enjoyed sitting among his peers as all their sins were exposed, but if the commissioners were not going to listen to him, perhaps they would respond when one of the most respected advocates for the treatment of the insane denounced them before the entire world.

To keep it constructive, Kirkbride announced that the Association wasn't going to get into how "the pauper lunatics of this community should have been allowed to lapse into that depth of degradation and neglect, of which, it would be difficult, elsewhere, to find a parallel." Instead, he made an "appeal to the authorities of this mighty and opulent metropolis of the Western world" to first abandon "those miserable apologies for insane hospitals, known as the old and the new madhouses," and go back to Alexander Jackson Davis's original design. Then do away with the practice of leaving inmates "to the tender mercies of thieves and prostitutes." Everyone from the attendants all the way up to the commissioners should be hired based on merit and not economy or political favors.

Nothing changed. It would only get much, much worse.

By the time the Rev. William Glenney French got to Blackwell's there were ten institutions on the Island, all of which were under the direction of a new department, created in 1860. Administratively, the new department wasn't a big change from the previous departments which oversaw the island, beginning with the commissioners of the Almshouse and Bridewell (the name of the prison downtown). Patients, convicts, and poor people were still managed by the same commissioners and they were still crowded together on the same narrow, two-mile-long island. Inmates of the Asylum continued to be locked up at night with convicts. The only real difference was the name of the new division, which clearly and alliteratively stated the relationship that everyone already believed naturally existed: the Department of Public Charities and Correction.

REV. FRENCH SPENT his first summer on Blackwell's getting the lay of the land by regularly walking the length of the island. Beginning at the northern end, he went from institution to institution, meeting with and listing all the Protestants on the island, whom he hoped to serve.

His first entries in what would be annual reports contained brief descriptions of each institution in the order in which he came upon them, beginning with the Lunatic Asylum, then the Workhouse, the Almshouse, the Penitentiary, and finally Charity Hospital. The Workhouse was where people convicted of minor crimes like vagrancy and intoxication were sent; the Almshouse was the city's "poorhouse"; and the Penitentiary was the city prison for people convicted of more serious crimes, usually with sentences of two years or less. Convicts with longer sentences were generally sent to places like Sing Sing, the State prison in Ossining, New York. There were exceptions however, and sometimes people who were convicted of murder were sent to the Penitentiary. Charity Hospital took care of the indigent poor.

French soon settled into his routine, traversing the entire Island daily, except Saturdays, his one day off. Years later, in one annual report he calculated that he'd "travelled on foot, on a low average, 3 miles a day," which had added up to 14,688 miles thus far.

From the ferry landing he'd head south, taking the river road, which ran along the convict-built sea wall to the Asylum. He was sometimes met and accompanied by Johnny the Horse, an inmate of the Island who'd been there since he was a young boy and who believed himself a horse. Curing insanity was still a relatively new concept and perhaps physicians didn't know where to begin with Johnny. He was harmless enough, however, and seemingly happy. With an unraveled rope functioning as a tail, he'd paw the ground like a horse, and deliver packages around the Island while hitched to a crude wooden soapbox-style cart. Johnny the Horse, whose real name was John Demorest, became a favorite Island "sight." Sadly, Demorest never did get better. He would live out his days in one institution after another, galloping around until he no longer could.

The Asylum itself sat opposite Seventy-Ninth to Eightieth Streets in Manhattan. The two islands lay so close to each other that inmates on Blackwell's could watch the ever-changing steel, brick, and granite panorama on the opposite shore. Commissioners would mention this in their reports as if the views of New York City were an entertaining feature, but in reality it was like being on the wrong side of a moat surrounding an enchanted, glittering palace.

Anyone entering the Asylum was immediately assaulted by the sights, sounds, and scents of daily institutional life. There was no proper reception or waiting room. The central and main administration building of the Asylum, the Octagon, was originally supposed to be merely a corner building, and so no physical entrance had been built. Instead, both visitors and inmates entered the Asylum through a door in the Octagon that led directly to the basement. Entering an insane asylum would have been under the best of circumstances an unnerving experience, but this arrangement took it straight to appalling. Noxious odors from the kitchen permeated the entire floor and before anyone had a chance to wonder why inmates were being fed food that smelled so sickening, their attention would be caught by whoever they passed on the stairs. On any given day that might be violent inmates, sick inmates, dead inmates as they were being carried out, "whole companies of firemen, soldiers, or excursion parties," or workers on their way to and from the kitchen, laundry, and elsewhere. Those workers, of course, might include convicts from the Workhouse or Penitentiary, or inmates from the Asylum itself. French would have seen what Dickens and Kirkbride had seen plus twenty-four years of further deterioration.

Even stout-hearted men must have crumbled. After Moses Ranney died from typhoid fever, Dr. Ralph Parsons took over and one of his first acts was to have the sewers and privies inspected to root out sources of the Island's health problems. They didn't yet know what caused typhoid fever, but they knew contaminated water was one means of transmission. What they found upon investigation was that waste had "gradually oozed through, saturating the woodwork of the floors and ceiling beneath, and, on the lower floor, forming cesspools, the stench arising," confirming that their economies had been, for some, a death sentence.

Mortality in the Asylum was an ongoing problem, and for many the Asylum itself was a death sentence. Conditions like overcrowding and malnourishment contributed to the causes of death most commonly listed: consumption (tuberculosis), phthisis pulmonalis (also tuberculosis), and diarrhea (likely the result of dysentery). Two other frequent determinations, "exhaustion from mania" and asthenia—a nervous condition characterized by loss of strength and physical weakness—each sound more like a description of symptoms than a true diagnosis or cause of death. Although they were seen as actual conditions then, a medical examiner today would look for an underlying cause. Scores of inmates were also carried off as a result of syphilis infections (the symptoms of which may have prompted their admission), and the occasional cholera outbreak, which would spread throughout the entire island.

The spread of disease was not the only danger of overcrowding. Parsons warned of the potential for violence when putting two patients in a room meant for one, but like Ranney before him, he was ignored. Cells throughout the Asylum were doubled up, which would eventually lead to just what Parsons feared.

The Lodge sat on the eastern side of the Island, not far from the main building, and like all the other buildings it was made from stone quarried on the Island. It was a small, three-story building with an attic and a basement. Each cell measured a mere five by twelve feet and was designed to hold one violent patient only.

But from the beginning they were doing all the things they'd said they'd never do, such as installing doors with small openings, like prison doors. To make matters more unlivable, all the cells in the Lodge were inside rooms, with no windows, another design they'd previously called inhumane. Into each of those tiny windowless cells, not even as wide as the average female arm span, would go two of the Asylum's most out-of-control patients, who were locked in together at 6 p.m. every night and not let out until the morning. With twenty-two cells on three floors, that put their capacity at sixty-six patients. By 1868, 190 women were housed in the Lodge (figures were not given for the men, but in general there were always more women in the Lodge; four halls were assigned to them and two were assigned to the men). The Lodge soon became known to all as the worst and most dangerous place in the Asylum.

On February 12, 1869, twenty-five-year-old Margaret McLaughlin, an Irish immigrant, was murdered by Catherine Shay in their cell at the Lodge. Shay had grabbed a small wooden tub, which functioned as a chamber pot, and brought it down on McLaughlin's head, fracturing her skull. Since screaming was not unusual in the Lodge, if any inmates had shrieked or called out for help they would have been ignored by the single watchman on duty. At five o'clock the next morning, nurse Eliza Dunnigan opened the door and found McLaughlin on the floor. She lived five more hours.

To ease the crowding, an Asylum for the Insane for the men was built on Wards Island, further north in the East River. By 1872, the Lunatic Asylum on Blackwell's was officially a woman's asylum, although some men were left behind to do the work the women could not.

Like everyone else, French would have entered the Asylum through the basement in the Octagon, and from there he would have made his way up to Hall 3. The chapel originally planned for one of the connecting buildings was never built. Instead, French was given space at one end of Hall 3, in the middle house in the main building. Hall 3 was the most presentable space in the Asylum. This was where inmates referred to as the "better class of patients" lived. When visitors from various committees came to inspect and report on the Asylum, they were taken here. Patients in Hall 3 were docile and generally convalescent, and were therefore the least disturbing. Visitors rarely saw the Lodge.

French did his best to fix up his designated corner in a "churchly manner," as he would note in an early report. He was allowed to install a chancel rail, to separate his makeshift altar from the congregation and passing inmates and workers, and to put up pictures and lay out altar linens.

French was hopeful at first, and he made do. But to see what Dickens saw not just once but day in and day out; to go "from one scene of suffering to another," threatened to overwhelm him. It wasn't long before his reports were peppered with lines like "No person can have an idea, until he sees it, of the degradation of the city poor."

The worst part was to see the suffering and feel powerless to really help. Ferrying back to the city every night was like exiting the battlefield of a war he could do nothing to end. He was only one man, with little money (and a wife and three young sons to support). He also couldn't say too much about what he saw. The Mission was there at the discretion of the Department of Public Charities and Correction, who could revoke their passes at any time (anyone who wasn't an employee of the city had to have a pass to be allowed on the Island). There was no chance of helping anyone if he wasn't there. So he would sit silently and bitterly on the ferry, writing lines like "To know the opportunities for good, and not be able to improve them . . ." His superiors would remind him that his mission was to provide spiritual support and consolation only, but even that was a challenge.

As the months passed, French learned to carve out time for services at each institution, and for private meetings with nurses and patients as needed. Sometimes he'd run errands in the city for inmates, like picking up paper and envelopes, or mailing the letters they wrote. He also made sure to go down to Printing House Square once a week to pick up newspapers that had been donated to the Island, keeping an eye out for German newspapers for the German inmates who could neither speak nor read English, and who regularly begged him for reading material in their native language.

Every Sunday morning he'd hold services in his corner of Hall 3, and look out at his congregants. The faces that looked back were in distinctly different states of recovery. Some were attentive, almost hungry with need, and they didn't miss a thing he said. But a certain percentage, he saw, were unreachable by words or reason. Something drew them to his services, likely an even more desperate need, but they sat like anesthetized puppets.

The "most painful feature of all," he wrote in his annual report, though, was simply witnessing daily "the sight of men and women, sitting around, hour after hour, with sad and hopeless faces . . . and leading this dull existence sometimes for years."

There was a fear among the general public that once you were confined to the Asylum you could be trapped there for years. Their fear was not unfounded. The 1874 annual report for the Department of Public Charities and Correction (written by the commissioners, and the wardens, physicians, and superintendents who ran the institutions) lists the following terms of residence for patients in the Lunatic Asylum, including twenty poor souls who were in there with no record of how long:

Five to ten years: 79
Ten to twenty years: 99
Twenty to thirty years: 93
Thirty to forty years: 12
Forty to fifty years: 3
Sixty to seventy years: 1
Lifetime: 84
Unknown: 20

A few years later, while testifying before a Senate committee looking into abuses at insane asylums, a young doctor would talk about how they'd found at least sixty patients without commitment papers or admission documents of any kind. "No one knew who had sent these patients to the asylum, and no record could be found."

As long as the Asylum was managed by the Department of Public Charities and Correction, lengthy commitments never went away. In 1893, the Department's last annual report in the nineteenth century, they listed 233 lifetime commitments.

Being confined to one small space for even relatively short commitments was stultifying, never mind for years, and French saw that the inmates of the Asylum were in great need of diversion. Moral treatment itself called for leisure activities. It was not therapeutic to have inmates sitting alone for long periods brooding on whatever distressed them, and superintendents would list their efforts to address the problem in a section of the annual report called Amusements. This might include lectures given by the medical staff, or concerts performed by musicians who would occasionally make the trip across the river. A big favorite, and one that caught the morbid fascination of journalists, was an event they called the Lunatics' Ball. On special holidays they'd fit up one of the pavilions as a dancing hall and everyone—patients, attendants, and doctors alike—would dance.

Perhaps the most beguiling form of entertainment offered were the captivating displays from a device called a magic lantern. A magic lantern was something like a slide show projector, but a skillful slide producer could create spectacles that seemed almost like a motion picture. After long stretches without a single distraction it was positively astounding to walk into a darkened room to see illustrations of a daring voyage to the Arctic or phantasmagorical images of goblins and ghosts glowing, sometimes appearing to dance, on the Asylum walls. Inmates were spellbound. But it wasn't a simple matter to get the apparatus there and to set it up. This was before electric light and the various methods of illumination that were open to them, like burning oil or gas, or oxyhydrogen light, which produced the brightest displays but was also extremely hot, had to be carefully managed. Inmates were lucky if they were treated to a handful of magic lantern performances a year.

Even if the Asylum managers came up with one amusement a week, that still left the inmates with a lot of time with little to do beyond dwelling on their dismal circumstances.

As French made his daily rounds and regularly confronted their staring faces, he once again felt impotent. He was just a humble priest, and as a Protestant he was a minority clergyman as well. While Protestants ruled in New York and America, on Blackwell's Island, where the Irish made up the greatest percentage of inmates, followed usually by Germans, Catholics were in the majority. What could one priest bring to entertain an average daily population of 7,000 people? His next idea may have come from those Catholic Germans, who due to the language barrier felt the most isolated of all. Whenever they saw him coming they would approach him with the same eager and consistent plea: Bring us something to read. Books were the one simple and relatively affordable form of entertainment within French's power to provide.

On one of his tours of the Island, French took stock of the libraries in each institution. There was a lot a "humble priest" could do, it turned out. The Penitentiary, the Workhouse, and Charity Hospital had none. The Almshouse had the modest beginnings of a library, and there was a library in the office of the resident physician of the Lunatic Asylum, but it was not truly accessible to patients. French's first step was to get permission to move the books out of the physician's office and into the hall where the patients could actually borrow them.

Next, he put out a call for books, newspapers, and magazines. He placed ads, put up flyers, and hit up all his friends and contacts. Like many librarians of his time, French would have preferred to provide reading geared towards self-improvement, and he looked down on novels as something frivolous. Back in 1839, in the *First Annual Report of the Board of Education*, someone wrote, "In the reports of some of the French hospitals for lunatics, the reading of romances is set down as one of the standing causes of insanity." But that was then and this was now, and if the inmates wanted novels, French would do his best to provide them. He also didn't forget the Germans and made a specific plea for books in their language. But only one person, Ernst Steiger, a German immigrant bookseller and publisher, responded.

In his first few years French established libraries in the institutions that had none, and continued to add to them, and to the libraries that were already there.

His ambitious project also added a new and crucial activity to his weekly routine. On Tuesdays, as he walked around the Island, he distributed books, newspapers, and other reading materials. It gave him the perfect opportunity to let new inmates know the libraries were there, but more importantly, it gave him a friendly way to get to know everyone, regardless of their beliefs. He became so trusted by inmates and managers alike that he was given a special key that opened every door in the Asylum. As a result, more than any other person before him who wasn't an employee, French got to see what life was really like for the inmates of the Asylum.

In May of 1872, the year French came to Blackwell's, there were 1,036 patients in the Asylum. Nine hundred thirty-seven of them were women and ninety-nine were men who'd been left behind to work. Most of them were Irish, temperate, meaning they didn't drink alcohol (self-reported), between twenty and forty years old, married (among the men, more were single), and they could read and write. They generally worked as housekeepers or domestics, and the most frequently applied diagnosis was "mania."

The most famous inmate in the Asylum in French's first year was the Irish nun Sister Mary Stanislaus, who was in the papers almost daily now as she and her lawyer, John D. Townsend, fought for her release. Townsend, who was thirty-seven years old at the time of Sister Mary's trial, was something of a celebrity himself. He was a risk taker who once thought he'd live his life on the sea, a career he began while still in his teens. By the time he reached twenty, he was a second mate on the fastest and most famous clipper ship at the time, the *Flying Cloud*. Later he inherited a bunch of money and ended up in law school after losing that inheritance in a failed investment. He then became the kind of lawyer who defended murderers, faced down Tweed-corrupted judges, and helped win freedom for people committed to New York asylums.

Stories of people locked up in insane asylums against their will have always held a particular fascination with the public, and the courtroom for Sister Mary's case was consistently packed with people who wanted to see if she was crazy, and if she wasn't, could Townsend successfully get her out.

SISTER MARY STANISLAUS

Committed to the Lunatic Asylum on Blackwell's Island
August 3, 1872
Diagnosis: Monomania

———◆———

O N MARCH 14, 1871, Sister Mary Stanislaus was staying at her sister Bridget's apartment at 8 East Eighteenth Street in Manhattan, when Bridget ran into Mary's bedroom crying. Eliza, their other sister, was dying, she sobbed, and they were leaving right then to see her. Sister Mary quickly put her private papers away and the two women boarded a streetcar to Central Park. When Bridget insisted on taking a carriage the rest of the way, Sister Mary felt the tiniest bit of alarm. It was only a short distance and they could have easily walked. Her instincts were correct. "Take a good look around you," Bridget announced as the carriage came to a stop at 116th Street and Tenth Avenue. "I won't deceive you any longer. This is an insane asylum."

If you had to be committed to a lunatic asylum, the Bloomingdale Asylum, where Bridget had taken her, was the place to be. When Bloomingdale first opened in 1821 it accepted all patients. Paupers were paid for by a grant from the state, and others were billed according to a sliding scale. Once the Asylum on Blackwell's was operational, however, only a small number of pauper patients were accepted at Bloomingdale, at the discretion of the Bloomingdale Board of Governors. The board at Bloomingdale still welcomed patients from working class families, who might be charged as little as $6 a week (the equivalent of a week's wages for many of the working class), while the families of the wealthy paid anywhere from $25 to $100 and occasionally more.

Bloomingdale Asylum became *the* destination asylum for the wealthy of New York. It didn't just have one library, it had several, which became progressively more refined as you moved to the quieter and fancier wards. In the most exclusive wards, oilcloths were replaced with carpets, the chairs were more plush, and the paintings hanging on the walls and the books on the shelves were more valuable. Bloomingdale also boasted a billiard room and lovely landscaped grounds which included a croquet court. While Blackwell's would admit thousands every year, the number of patients at Bloomingdale generally did not exceed 300.

SISTER MARY REFUSED to leave the carriage. Dr. Dwight Burrell, the assistant physician, came out and asked her gently, "Did not you say you were going to kill yourself?" Two physicians who had visited her at her sister's had already signed affidavits saying that she had. Their statements were then taken to a police justice who immediately signed a lunacy warrant for her commitment.

"I never said any such thing," Sister Mary insisted. But living in her sister's home was far from ideal, and relations between the sisters were severely strained. She may have taken in the large federal style brownstone which looked more like a mansion, and the elegant landscaping by Frederick Law Olmsted and Calvert Vaux, the designers of Central Park, and thought, *Maybe I'd be happier there.* Sister Mary left the carriage and entered the asylum. It would become her home for the next seventeen months.

Sister Mary's initial descriptions of her experiences at Bloomingdale were mostly positive, but she did not accept her diagnosis and often begged to be sent to "the Island." Although there are several islands around Manhattan, whenever anyone said "the Island" it was understood that they meant Blackwell's. Sister Mary must have known that the Asylum for paupers on Blackwell's would be a step down from the genteel Bloomingdale. But she saw the Island as her only hope. There was a priest there, she believed, who would help her get in touch with the Archbishop of Halifax, who she was sure would rescue her.

The Archbishop of Halifax had recruited Sister Mary in 1854, when he was still the Bishop Thomas Louis Connolly, and she was Rose McCabe, a twenty-three-year-old Irish immigrant living in a convent in downtown Manhattan. Connolly came to New York looking for novices for a new order of sisters, and he had no trouble interesting the young Rose in a mission to care for Irish orphans in Canada. Rose left New York City for New Brunswick, where she took her vows and became Sister Mary Stanislaus, of the Sisters of Charity.

Things went well for the next few years, as she helped establish missions around New Brunswick. Then in 1861 she unexpectedly took two postulants with her and defected to Bishop James Rogers in Chatham, where she wanted to start a school. That uproar might have passed but Sister Mary wouldn't stop telling anyone who would listen about her "suffering and persecution" at the hands of Mother Vincent, the superioress back at the convent she'd fled. She made Mother Vincent out to be some kind of queen of the mean girls who got all the novices to insult her and freeze her out. Connolly counseled patience and asked that everyone be kind to Sister Mary.

It wasn't long before relations between Sister Mary and Bishop Rogers also soured; he described her as "a whimsical, discontented, impractical creature, unhappy herself and rendering everyone around her unhappy also." Sister Mary soon took off yet again. When Mother Vincent refused to take her back, Bishop John Sweeney had her put on a boat back to the states, where over the next ten years she taught school in Auburn, New York, and New York City, and spent time as a resident in an almshouse in Brooklyn as well.

It's not clear what Sister Mary thought the Archbishop of Halifax would do for her after she left on such bad terms. There'd been no contact between them in the ten years since. But in the summer of 1872 Sister Mary did make a very useful friend at Bloomingdale, Jasper T. Van Vleck. Van Vleck was a former Wall Street banker who'd been dragged from his breakfast table and committed to the Bloomingdale Asylum a couple of weeks after Sister Mary's arrival. The quiet, penniless nun brought out Van Vleck's protective instincts and when he hired the prominent criminal lawyer John D. Townsend to get him out the following summer, he instructed Townsend to secure Sister Mary's release as well.

Townsend went to court and a writ of habeas corpus was issued on August 3, ordering the Bloomingdale Asylum to produce Sister Mary in court on August 6. The managers of Bloomingdale must have caught wind of what was happening, because on August 3, one of the city commissioners who oversaw all New York's public charitable institutions met with Police Justice John McQuade of the Fifth District. A new warrant of commitment for insanity was issued for Sister Mary, this time to Blackwell's Island. On Blackwell's, Sister Mary would no longer be Bloomingdale's responsibility or problem (and the Bloomingdale managers were now, presumably, in debt to that commissioner).

Two months after committing Sister Mary, Justice McQuade, an associate of William M. "Boss" Tweed—the powerful leader of Tammany Hall, the notoriously corrupt political organization—was called before a Senate investigating committee. They wanted him to explain some bills he'd okayed for materials and work for the Harlem Courthouse. No one could verify that the materials were ever either received or the work completed, and what did he have to say about that? Although he wasn't indicted and tried, McQuade never held a public office again. Tweed would be sent to the Island the following year.

Sister Mary had gotten her wish. They had her on a ferry to the Island that very day. Like Rev. French on his first trip there, she would have steamed towards Blackwell's full of hope and anticipation. Van Vleck had Townsend on the case, and soon she'd be able to look for the priest who would help her get back in touch with the Archbishop. After being dropped off at the guardhouse and escorted to the New York City Lunatic Asylum, Sister Mary must have believed it wouldn't be long before she was free.

SISTER MARY STANISLAUS
IS ADMITTED INTO THE ASYLUM

———◆———

IDEALLY, WHEN A new patient arrived at the Asylum a history would be taken by one of the assistant physicians. This would include anything that was known about what brought the person there, the patient's own account of themselves, and the results from a medical exam. They'd note Sister Mary's age, height, weight, the color of her eyes, where she was born, her religion, marital status, occupation, the occupation of her parents, whether or not she was a drinker, and if she could read or write.

Based on this examination she would be assigned to one of four classes of patients. The loudest and most violent were Class One. "Idiots" and the epileptic were Class Two. People with an intellectual disability were called idiots in the nineteenth century, and epilepsy was not only considered a form of insanity, epileptics were separated from the "ordinary insane" because they were thought to be prone to violence and criminal acts and were, overall, a very "unpromising class of patients." Class Three was the most hopeful category. This was the designation for patients who were considered convalescent and improving. Finally, Class Four was where they put patients who were in an intermediate stage, and this included incurables who were deemed harmless and "not possessed of bad habits." "Bad" or what were also frequently referred to as "filthy" habits usually meant masturbation, or playing with feces.

Moral treatment dictated that the different classes of patients be kept apart. "The indiscriminate mingling of the mild and furious, clean and filthy, convalescent and idiotic, need only be witnessed to be deprecated," Dr. Macdonald wrote in the original plan.

This did not work well in practice. The fact that the Asylum was "crowded beyond the bounds of humanity" made it impossible. Patients were put where there was room. Another big problem was assistant physician turnover. The job didn't pay well. It's not surprising that as soon as young physicians gained enough experience to be effective they moved on to higher-paying positions elsewhere. It was so hard to find people to even take the job that sometimes undergraduates were hired. Patients were essentially being classified by trainees.

According to annual reports, after whatever constituted classification, Sister Mary would then have been given a warm bath and a change of clothes. This was another instance where reality did not match good intentions. Where there were stoves to heat the water they weren't always working and when there was no way to heat water it was carried over from other buildings in pails. This was a time-consuming and grueling chore. Compounding the problem was the fact that in the bathrooms, "The water flows slowly and is limited in supply," Ralph L. Parsons, the Asylum's resident physician, wrote in the 1867 annual report. "If the water be changed for each new bather much time and a large amount of water are required, and the supply of hot water is liable to fail. Consequently it is not found practicable to change the water for each new bather."

Bathing all the patients in the same bathwater became standard practice. This is even more repugnant then it might initially sound. If all the women were relatively healthy and clean it might have been merely disgusting. But one or two of the women who'd gotten into the water may have been playing with their feces. Another may have had lice, another open sores from syphilis. The water would be reused and reused until it became more sludge than water, and women would have to step into water that was brown and oily, with floating bits of waste and vermin. No one wanted to get into that. Attendants would have to be called, who just as often as not were convicts from the Workhouse, and bath time was rarely the calming experience planners imagined. Afterwards, patients were dried off with the same towels that might have just been used to dry a patient with an unidentified illness.

Going to the bathroom was almost as revolting. The toilets were a long trough covered by wooden seats and filled with water. There was a plug that was supposed to be regularly pulled in order to drain the water through a sewer into the river, but like everything else, that wasn't done according to the prescribed schedule and a suffocating odor usually permeated the area.

The clothing given to patients following their baths was poorly made, rarely fit, and was never enough against the elements. A reporter who visited in December one year wrote that many in the Asylum were severely underdressed to face a New York winter, and their feet were purple from the cold.

On her first night on Blackwell's, Sister Mary would have been supplied with one thin blanket and put wherever there was a spare straw mattress, which was likely on the floor, wedged between the wall and the lucky patient who got the one bed. They didn't have gas throughout the Asylum yet, and oil lamps were only given to attendants, so Sister Mary would have gone to bed at sunset, and the door to her room locked.

Her name would be added to the prescription book that was kept in every ward and hall. This book listed the number of patients in that hall, the names of any new patients since the previous day, how many were sick and how many were able to work, and the names of anyone who had recently died. In addition to instructions for medications, if there were any special orders for any of the patients those would be noted here as well. If no medications were indicated for Sister Mary when she was admitted, they would wait a few days before deciding what to prescribe.

The prescription book also listed how many patients in the ward were currently in restraints. Under the guidelines of moral treatment, restraints were not to be used except in the most violent cases in order "to control destructive, homicidal and suicidal propensities." Restraints used in the

Lunatic Asylum on Blackwell's Island included belting inmates to a chair, wristlets, and camisoles, which was another name for a straitjacket, and described by a doctor as "a garment very much like a bag with sleeves. . . . The ends of the sleeves are tied behind the patient, fastening the arms behind—more or less cramped." Another common restraining device were the innocent-sounding muffs. "The hands of the patient are within the muff," a doctor described, "with the ends strapped around the elbow, and body besides, so that the patient cannot use his hands, to keep him from breaking windows and masturbating and so on."

The most disturbing method of restraint of all was a device called a crib. These were essentially tiny horizontal cages, and were only used at night, they claimed. The patient would be laid down inside, the top would be brought down and locked, and there they would remain until morning. Many objected to them, including Dr. Edward C. Spitzka, a noted neurologist who would later describe how "an excitable person will squirm in it like a squirrel."

In their 1858 annual report the commissioners claimed that all forms of restraint had been removed from the Lunatic Asylum. In the 1862 report, Moses Ranney said that they were using few restraints, but never iron wristlets and leg-locks, so it seems unlikely that they were ever completely gone. Eventually, they gave up all pretense and started keeping a separate restraint book, to list how often they were resorting to these measures. In 1882, for instance, 351 women were restrained 3,086 times. "Insane women on the whole are more unmanageable than are insane men," one superintendent wrote, defending the practice. Chemical restraints like morphine and opium were also often employed, but their use was rarely reported as such. Instead, Asylum managers would emphasize the curative and therapeutic benefits of their application.

Sister Mary would have been kept inside until they had a better sense of her. If she was unlucky she would be assigned to cleaning the halls and the putrid bathrooms. If luck was on her side, however, and she was deemed a quiet or convalescent patient, they would assign her a pleasant activity, like sewing or knitting. And, if it was not currently being used as a dormitory, she would have been allowed to visit the Amusement Hall whenever activities like the magic lantern were scheduled.

Eventually Sister Mary would be permitted to go on supervised walks with other patients. For years only the tamer patients had the privilege of joining these outside strolls. Patients from the Lodge kept bolting straight for the East River the first chance they got, occasionally disappearing beneath the dark brown waters before anyone could attempt to save them. Would-be rescuers sometimes died trying. Nicknamed "river runners," some of these inmates were just trying to get away; the island of Manhattan was so tantalizingly close. Any decent swimmer unaware of the currents would look across and think, *Surely I could make that.* (No record of anyone from the Asylum having made it could be found, but on rare occasions men from the Penitentiary or Workhouse managed to reach the other shore alive.) Others, who had enough of the baths, and being roughed up by attendants, or locked inside a crib in a dark, windowless room, saw death in the river as an acceptable means of escape. Outside became off-limits for the women in the Lodge.

One of the medical superintendents would later come up with a scheme to allow the more difficult patients to walk again in the sunshine. He called his design a "wagon procession." He built a small wagon, painted it in bright colors, and attached a long rope, also painted in the same gaudy colors. Spaced along the rope were smaller ropes with rings on the end. Patients would walk along the rope two abreast, with colored and flowing scarves tied around their waists to hide the leather belts which locked them to the rings. The scarves were there to preserve the inmates' dignity, the superintendent explained. But they were also there to avoid alarming visitors, who wouldn't see the belts and locks, and instead view the sight as a happy, holiday-like parade. During each stroll, a crippled or injured patient was given the honor of riding at the head of the procession in the wagon.

Sister Mary Stanislaus arrived on Blackwell's in the summer of 1872, just as it was entering one of the most crowded and lethal periods in the

Island's history. Despite their precautions, the Lunatic Asylum was the deadliest institution on Blackwell's Island. Out of the 2,023 treated the year before, 171 died in the Asylum. That put their mortality rate at around 8.5 percent. The only years with more deaths were 1849, 1854, and 1866, when there were cholera outbreaks. In comparison, the Penitentiary, with a population of 2,386, who were certainly a more violent lot, had only ten deaths. The Workhouse, also a house of correction, where 21,882 drunkards, vagrants, and disorderly persons of all stripes were sentenced, had 110 deaths, or a mere 0.5 percent. The Almshouse, with 3,716 inmates who were mostly old and sick women, had 73 fatalities. Even Charity Hospital, filled with many of the sickest, poorest people in New York City, had a lower mortality rate.

A large part of the problem was financial. The amount spent every week per patient in 1874, $1.62, was the lowest of all asylums in the state, the country, and the rest of the world. Even the criminally insane got more. Generally $4.00 a week was spent on the inmates of the New York State Asylum for Insane Criminals in Auburn. At a time when many people thought African Americans were less than human, more went towards their care. The Central Lunatic Asylum for the Colored Insane in Virginia spent $3.79. A reporter who visited the Asylum in 1869 wrote that the patients were being slowly starved to death. Although the commissioners claimed the diet had been fixed, how fixed could it be, the reporter asked, when only 13 cents a day was being spent to feed them?

To make matters worse, Sister Mary Stanislaus walked into this dangerous realm with three strikes against her. Women were already considered more difficult to handle, but in addition to being a member of the crazier gender, Sister Mary was Irish and a Catholic. The commissioners (and many other Americans) were convinced that other countries were sending their undesirables here, palming off their care on the United States. Of these castoffs, the lowest of the low were the Irish. Although they took the jobs no one else wanted, they were seen as job-stealers, and anti-immigrant groups like the Know-Nothing Party targeted them for the worst of their abuse. Some asylums even had separate Irish wards. The Irish also practiced a religion which Protestant physicians and staff found "particularly depraved and offensive," according to Lynn Gamwell and Nancy Tomes in *Madness in America*. Sister Mary, with her brogue and the nun's habit that she never stopped wearing, would have borne the weight of all that prejudice, and the idea that the money, as little as it was, was being spent on people who should be someone else's problem.

Dr. Moses Ranney had a sympathetic view of the shock and disappointment immigrants felt when arriving in the glittering city. In a *Harper's Weekly* article he described his female patients as "immigrant girls (chiefly Irish) who had been deluded, seduced, cheated and otherwise ill-used on arrival here; and who, on realizing their miserable condition, had gone mad from the shock of disappointment."

Dr. Parsons, still the resident physician at the time of Sister Mary's arrival, described the Irish as people "of exceptionably bad habits" whose chances for recovery were not good. In a paper, Parsons claimed that "the majority of our Irish patients are of a low order of intelligence, and very many of them have imperfectly developed brains. When such persons become insane, I am inclined to think that the prognosis is unfavorable."

Although Sister Mary thought Blackwell's would lead to her salvation, she quickly saw how wrong she'd been.

The Rev. French, who had arrived on Blackwell's just a few months before, met Sister Mary on one of his routine visits, in which he would seek out and introduce himself to new patients. Although French envied the Catholics their influence—they had the best chapels in all the institutions on the Island—he was as kind to them as he was to anyone else.

The two hit it off. After their first meeting French called on Sister Mary regularly. Sometimes she'd close the door when he came into her cell. People are watching me, she told him. That does sound a little crazy and paranoid, but it was true. Being alone with a female patient behind closed doors wouldn't do, however, and French would always open the door, telling her they weren't going to be saying anything that couldn't be overheard by all.

One Sunday morning when French went to visit her, Sister Mary's room was empty. He found a nurse who called to an attendant, and together they went down a hall to a room he'd never seen before. He peered inside when they unlocked the door, but it was too dark. Sister Mary emerged from the lightless room with her dress torn and a chunk of her hair missing. Why had she been shut up like that? The woman in the room next to her had started crying out the night before, Sister Mary told him. When she called to the nurse to help the woman, the nurse, who was angry at being forced to leave her bed, had an attendant drag Sister Mary out of her room instead. They locked her up in this filthy room, where she would have remained for who knows how long if French hadn't insisted they produce her. The other woman was left to scream out unanswered.

French, who was now well aware of how things operated on Blackwell's Island, knew the nurse in question. He would later describe her as a tyrannical and very cruel woman. The idea that she would punish a patient for simply asking for help for another was entirely plausible, especially if the nurse had been woken from a sound sleep. French also knew that when it came to conflicting accounts of what happened in the wards when the doctors were not around, the nurses' and attendants' versions of events were always accepted over the patients'. No one would take Sister Mary's word for anything. When he turned to Sister Mary and made it clear that he believed her and was on her side, the comfort she felt must have been enormous. French wanted to offer more than his faith, and told his superiors about what was going on, with the understanding that they would take his concerns to the commissioners. But nothing seemed to change.

Fortunately, Jasper T. Van Vleck, Sister Mary's protector, had not forgotten her. His lawyer, John D. Townsend, filed a second writ of habeas corpus, compelling the commissioners to bring Sister Mary before Judge George C. Barrett of the New York Supreme Court on August 13. At least in Barrett's court Sister Mary wouldn't be subjected to the prevailing anti-Irish, anti-Catholic viewpoint. Born in Dublin, Judge Barrett was not only an Irish immigrant himself, he was the son of a clergyman.

THE TRIAL OF SISTER MARY

———◆———

S HE WOULD BECOME known as "the lunatic nun." Reporters who had written about Van Vleck's success at getting
out of Bloomingdale learned of Sister Mary's fight to get
out of Blackwell's, and once the papers got a hold of her story they didn't
let go. The lurid and newspaper-selling tales they sometimes told of sane
people committed to the lunatic asylum weren't always tales. In his book
Social Order/Mental Disorder, Andrew Scull, a professor at the University
of California at San Diego, writes what could describe Sister Mary's sister
Bridget: "The asylum provided a convenient and culturally legitimate alternative to coping with 'intolerable' individuals within the family."

The Asylum administrators themselves conceded that sane people were
occasionally wrongfully committed, although they claimed that they were
the ones to discover them. They sometimes included descriptions of their
cases in their annual reports under the heading *Improper Subjects*. Improper subjects, they said, were often "suffering temporary consequences
of recent debauch," which couldn't be properly sorted out until the woman
sobered up. Harriet Osborne, for instance, "a person of very limited education and dull of comprehension," turned out to be a laudanum addict.

Dr. Parsons unwittingly escalated interest in Sister Mary and suspicion
towards the Asylum when he refused to allow the reporters who'd rowed

over to the Island to see her and question her. All the local papers, the *New York Times*, *The Sun*, *The World*, the *New York Herald*, the *New-York Tribune*, and others were competing for coverage (and readers) and the public was dying to get the first look at the lunatic nun. Anyone who didn't have to be at work that Tuesday, August 13, 1872, jammed into every available spot in the Chambers Street courtroom. Which meant Sister Mary's fate would be witnessed by the press, high society, and the unemployed.

Her first appearance in court was brief. The *Boston Globe* wrote that "there is a wild, hungry, yearning look in her eyes, which is supposed to be characteristic of lunacy," although the reporter acknowledged this could also be because she'd been unjustly locked up in a place that might be as bad as it was rumored to be.

Court adjourned early to give Justice Barrett time to consider Townsend's opening argument that, according to an 1842 statute, committing Sister Mary based on a warrant signed by a police justice was improper. Sister Mary was sent back to the Lunatic Asylum where every day held the possibility of danger. Fewer people were dying that year, but that was only because they'd moved most of the men to the new asylum on Wards Island and there weren't as many people in the Asylum on Blackwell's. The number of women who died in 1872, ninety-two, was only four less than the year before.

While all this was going on, the *New-York Tribune* quietly assigned a young reporter named Julius Chambers to get himself committed to the Bloomingdale Asylum in order to report undercover on conditions. Chambers had prearranged his release with John Townsend, the same lawyer representing Sister Mary, to take place ten days after his commitment. The day after Sister Mary appeared in court for the first time, Julius Chambers entered the Bloomingdale Asylum.

Sister Mary's hopes for relief from a sympathetic judge were quickly quashed. Judge Barrett's involvement with the case was over at the end of August, when Barrett ruled that revised statutes in 1860 allowed for police justices to issue warrants for commitment, and that the 1842 statute

Townsend had cited applied to the State Lunatic Asylum at Utica alone. The only thing to be decided now was whether or not Sister Mary was insane. The case would resume the following Tuesday, on September 3, but with a different judge, William H. Leonard.

Leonard was briefly filling a vacancy left by Albert Cardozo, a judge in the pocket of Boss Tweed. Cardozo had resigned in order to avoid impeachment. Once again, Townsend must have felt things were going their way. Cardozo, who would have presided, considered Townsend his sworn enemy. It began a couple of years before, when Townsend defended two women Cardozo had sent to prison at the request of yet another magistrate who was a member of what was called Tweed's Ring. "You need never expect any favors from me as long as I'm on the bench," Cardozo promised. Judge Leonard would certainly be a friendlier adjudicator.

At ten o'clock in the morning on September 3, the courtroom was once again jammed with spectators. This was the day Sister Mary would finally get to tell her story in open court. Among the people filling the seats were two inmates recently released from the Bloomingdale Asylum; Sister Mary's friend and protector Jasper T. Van Vleck; and the young reporter Julius Chambers, who was now out of the Bloomingdale Asylum and in the process of writing his account for the *Tribune*. One newspaper noted that the crowd was mostly female. The women may have recognized that they could be in Sister Mary's shoes someday. According to Ellen Dwyer in her article "Civil Commitment Laws in Nineteenth-Century New York," "Increasingly vulnerable to commitment proceeding were the economically marginal, particularly if female, whose behavior had become strange and disturbing."

Judge Leonard opened the proceedings by saying that he didn't feel qualified to make a ruling about anyone's sanity and he wanted medical experts to testify. But we can't afford experts, Townsend immediately responded. Judge Leonard had no choice. With a reluctance so enormous it was obvious to everyone in the courtroom—reporters later commented on it—he allowed Sister Mary to take the stand.

As usual, Sister Mary was dressed in the plain, brown habit of the order of the Sisters of Charity. The *New York Herald* described her as a "small, delicate figure," who "appears much younger" than her years. (She was forty-one.) And when she spoke she had "a pleasing subdued expression, while an air of calm and majestic serenity mantles her pale features."

"I was baptized Rosa McCabe; my other name is Sister Mary Stanislaus Theresa," she began (Sister Mary, and others, used the names *Rose* and *Rosa* interchangeably). She told of being tricked with the story of a dying sister in order to get her to the Bloomingdale Asylum, where things were all right until she complained to the doctors about a nurse who had been abusing another patient. The doctors didn't believe her and the nurse later beat her. Like the nurses on Blackwell's, apparently, "Lizzie Riley could do what she liked," Sister Mary claimed.

Judge Leonard questioned her at length about her past, and she talked about leaving her missionary work in Canada due to a misunderstanding with Bishop Sweeney. All the young nuns insulted her there, but even though she was the injured party, she was the one compelled to leave. From there she went to Auburn, New York, to help found a convent, then to a nunnery in Baltimore, and finally to New York City, where she was ill-treated by her sister Bridget, who threw out her valuable papers and letters.

"What right have you to wear that dress?" John McKeon, the lawyer representing Bridget asked.

"It was given to me by competent church authority."

"Have you the right to wear it now?"

"Yes."

It was not an idle question. When she was sent back to the States in 1862, Bishop Sweeney dispensed Sister Mary from her vows. At that point she was no longer a nun and she wasn't a Sister of Charity. Wearing a habit was, at the very least, odd. She could have taken vows elsewhere, except she continued to call herself a Sister of Charity.

"Don't you recollect that a priest and a doctor planned to poison you in Thirty-Fifth Street," McKeon asked. It was another key point: her belief that there was a conspiracy to poison her convinced the doctors to sign the certificate for commitment. "I never intimated any such thing," she insisted. But then she made a rather damaging claim. It was Dr. Parsons, and not herself, who had said that a Father McAleer had tried to kill her. At this point it was four o'clock in the afternoon and Sister Mary had testified for three hours. Court was adjourned.

The next day the court heard from Drs. Bradford and Burdick, the men who had declared Sister Mary insane and had her committed to Blooming-dale. Both testified that Sister Mary said the Church was conspiring to poison her and to get her committed. She had even showed Bradford the alleged lethal powders, but Sister Mary's lawyer never asked him if he had made any attempt to identify the powder. Bradford also testified that she tried to interest him in the papers which gave her the right to be a nun, but once again Townsend didn't ask him about their contents or authenticity.

It was not a good day for Sister Mary. On one visit, Dr. Bradford told them, she had a bandage on her hand, claiming her sister had bitten her. When Bradford removed the cloth, however, there were no marks. Dr. Burdick mentioned a priest that Sister Mary had said made improper advances towards her when she was living on Thirty-Fifth street. She escaped his overtures by putting furniture against the door and climbing out a window. "I came to the conclusion that she was not altogether sound of mind; her eyes had a wild, staring expression, and were very restless in their sockets, such as is shown in persons laboring under great fear." The people in the courtroom may have squirmed uncomfortably at those remarks. Not only did the general public believe sane people were committed all the time, here was confirmation that it could happen simply by having the wrong look in your eye. Those fears may have become further entrenched when another doctor said one of the reasons he thought Sister Mary was insane was her "rolling of the eyes," and Dr. Parsons, who was in charge of the entire Asylum, said he determined her insanity by the expression of her face and the appearance of her eyes.

The next day the courtroom was once again filled to capacity. Townsend began his cross-examination of Dr. Burdick by asking if he recognized what Sister Mary was wearing. "I know nothing about the garb of the Roman Catholic Church," he answered gruffly, perhaps betraying his feelings towards the religion and a bias against Sister Mary. When Townsend then asked him to state everything he could remember Sister Mary saying, McKeon loudly objected. We heard all this yesterday, he complained to the judge.

Judge Leonard sustained McKeon's objection, and went even further. He announced that he'd decided that Sister Mary was a monomaniac, and she was better off in the Asylum. Monomania was a very general and popular diagnosis in the nineteenth century. It meant that the person was fixated on something to the point of madness.

Townsend jumped up, flabbergasted. "As your honor has prejudged the case, I will retire from it."

McKeon responded, and "very coolly," according to the *New York Herald*. "I move to dismiss the writ." He also invited Townsend to drop his complaint that there was any conspiracy to send Sister Mary to the Lunatic Asylum.

"I am not called on to answer," Townsend replied.

"I insist on an answer."

"I decline to answer."

"It is all humbuggery, and has been so from the beginning to the end, and had better stop at once."

Like that, it was over. Sister Mary could barely speak, and she turned in horror to her friend Van Vleck. "It will be all right my dear," he said to comfort her, "keep up a good heart." Townsend rushed over to explain that he was withdrawing so they could bring her case in front of another judge. Before the day was out Townsend issued a statement to the press. After briefly explaining what led to McKeon's objection when Townsend started cross-examining Dr. Burdick, he wrote, "In deciding the question against me, Judge Leonard took occasion to say that he had read the doctor's statement in a newspaper, and that when he saw Miss McCabe on the witness stand his impression was that she was a monomaniac. . . . No evidence whatever had been introduced to disprove the statements of Miss Rosa McCabe. . . . I shall apply for a writ to some other judge, who can wait until the evidence is produced before he expresses at least his opinion."

Another writ was issued and the crowds returned on October 28, before a young judge named John Sedgwick. Women were once again in the majority in the courtroom.

The lawyer representing the commissioners of the Department of Public Charities and Correction began by asking for a postponement and Townsend urgently objected. Sister Mary had been transferred to a vermin-infested ward containing the most violent inmates in the Asylum. A rat had run across her room right in front of him on the day he visited. Along with the agitated patients who screamed all night long, they made sleep or rest of any kind impossible. But neither the rats nor the screaming were the most pressing reasons for Townsend's apprehension. The door to their room had been ajar when he visited and he had overhead a Dr. Taylor ask an attendant, "Can't you get along without beating patients in this way?" If nothing else, would the judge allow Sister Mary to stay in his own house until her next court date?

But Judge Sedgwick refused to believe that this was what life was like in the Asylum. "I will make my own affidavit in the case," Townsend insisted. "I cannot assume such a state of facts," the judge answered. The next trial date was set for Friday, November 1. Sister Mary would remain where she was.

"Of course I must submit to the decision of the court," Townsend responded. "One thing is very certain, however, that if Miss McCabe is not now crazy she soon will be if she is much longer kept amid her present surroundings."

Sister Mary still had her wits about her when she took the stand at the beginning of November. "A sweeter and more plaintive voice is seldom heard," wrote the *New York Herald*. The court also finally heard from people who told a very different story from the one they'd heard so far.

Attendants from both Bloomingdale and Blackwell's testified that Sister Mary was a completely amiable patient who never showed a single sign of insanity. Dr. James H. Johnson from Blackwell's agreed. Yes, she gets excited sometimes when trying to make herself understood, he conceded, but she is not insane. Even more damning, a Dr. Nugent said he was asked by a Dr. McMahon to sign a certificate attesting to Sister Mary's insanity without having ever met her.

But then the expert witness for the Department of Public Charities and Correction, Dr. George Choate, took the stand. Although Choate based his diagnosis on a single one hour meeting, he was well known and respected in the field. He was the founder of a private sanatorium called Choate House, where *New-York Tribune* editor Horace Greeley would die just a few weeks later on November 29. Among the stories she told him, Choate testified, was one about asking Dr. Parsons to remove an injured toenail. According to Sister Mary, Parsons responded by saying he would like to pull out her tongue. Choate concluded that she was "morbidly suspicious," and had a "mild case of mania with delusions."

In spite of this, the next day started out more promisingly. Another doctor testified that Dr. McMahon had pressured him to sign a certificate declaring Sister Mary insane without having met her. Unlike the previous doctor, however, he didn't have a problem with that. When that wasn't enough to get her committed, Dr. McMahon asked him to meet with her and sign another. McMahon assured him he'd be well paid for his efforts. He agreed, but then refused to sign when he met with Sister Mary and found her perfectly sane.

Spectators in the courtroom woke up in a way they hadn't before when Father Michael McAleer, of the Church of St. Columba and the "improper advances," took the stand. McAleer had a commanding presence, and all the papers commented on his calm and authoritative demeanor. No, he never made improper advances towards Sister Mary, he testified, and, yes, he put her out of the house when she made this outrageous claim, but he didn't employ violence of any kind to do so.

Father Brady, a young priest who worked for him at the time and who was there, told a slightly different story. The trouble began when Father McAleer asked Sister Mary why she continued to wear her habit. She responded by accusing him of improper conduct. According to Brady, Father McAleer did not strike her or kick her, but her ousting wasn't exactly peaceful. Father McAleer jumped up, then took Sister Mary by the shoulders and rushed her to the door. She may have fallen to her knees at some point, Brady admitted. Sister Mary spoke up quietly at this point and said that Brady's account was accurate.

Father Brady also told the court that Sister Mary had come to him before this with stories of persecution and mistreatment by Father McAleer, but she talked so fast and indistinctly he had trouble understanding her. She also asked him to use his influence with the pastor at Auburn, "to allow her to wear her dress and still go out in the world and teach."

It's difficult to sort out the truth now, more than a century later. Sister Mary does seem to assume everyone was against her. But in some cases, they most assuredly were. It is not inconceivable, for instance, that Dr. Parsons, who believed women were hard to manage—particularly Irish women—might very well have snapped at her, especially at the end of a long day, and if Sister Mary was talking in the excited way that Dr. Johnson described.

Sister Mary believed her sister was conspiring to put her in an asylum, which of course was true, and she was also afraid that her sister would one day destroy her papers. On November 9, when the case resumed, Bridget was questioned about these papers. Sister Mary had often "expressed fear at their loss," she said, but the doctors had advised against sending them to her. What did she did do with them, she was asked. She destroyed them. Even though she was well aware of how important they were to Sister Mary, she said she did it "supposing they were of no account." It's an act of casual cruelty and indifference that is hard to understand.

Dr. Johnson, who believed her sane, gave an example of a seemingly insane story that turned out to be at least partially true. One day when he met with her she told him that Miss Goodwin's room (the matron of the Asylum) had a table set for four visitors. She said she suspected the table had been set for four priests who were plotting against her. That sounds completely delusional. But shortly thereafter he came across four priests in the corridor. That doesn't corroborate her story, of course; he didn't question them, yet four priests walking the wards of the Asylum was not a common sight. They could have come to advise Miss Goodwin about, among other things, Sister Mary, and it's at least somewhat understandable that Sister Mary didn't believe that advice would be in her best interests, even if it was.

Dr. Parsons, when trying to explain how he could find her insane when his colleague, Dr. Johnson, found her sane, said that if everything she said was true, she "showed much less feeling on the subject than a sane person would." In other words, she wasn't acting crazy enough.

There also seemed to be an assumption at the time that priests would never lie, and the idea that any of them could have behaved improperly towards her was simply outrageous. The fact that Sister Mary continued to call herself a Sister of Charity and wear a habit when she was no longer a nun does indicate a problem. But insanity, even in nineteenth-century terms?

Court convened a few more times. Dr. Johnson once again insisted Sister Mary was not insane, but eccentric, and, echoing Townsend's fear, that her eccentricity had been "magnified" by the "persecutions and privations to which the patient has been subjected."

The lawyers made their closing statements on November 21, and Judge Sedgwick announced his decision on December 17. Ultimately, he was convinced by Dr. Choate, who'd met with Sister Mary for an hour. Sedgwick concluded that she was insane, but curable, "if she can get the benefit of measures taken by skilled men in such cases."

Sister Mary would remain in the Lunatic Asylum until the following summer when Dr. Parsons let her out on a thirty-day pass. Thirty-day passes were occasionally granted to patients showing great improvement. At the end of the month, if all went well, and friends and family confirmed that improvement continued, the inmate would be discharged.

After staying first with a friend, Sister Mary returned to her sister Bridget's apartment. It didn't go any better than the last time, and Sister Mary reached out once more to John D. Townsend for aid. Townsend offered to take her in until they found a more permanent arrangement, but Bridget refused to allow it and Townsend wasn't sure how to proceed from there. He found out later that Sister Mary had gone to live with her old friend from Blackwell's, the Reverend French, and that she was very happy with French and his family. In the meantime, Townsend wrote to the Archbishop of Halifax, asking if the "Church did not feel itself bound to protect" her. He never heard back.

At the end of Sister Mary's thirty-day pass, Dr. Parsons pronounced "the lunatic nun" sane and she was formally discharged. Sister Mary hoped to make a living writing and selling a pamphlet of her life story, but what she really wanted was to be able to return to "her true vocation," according to a *New York Times* article, "devoting herself to the poor and needy."

That year the state would create the office of State Commissioner in Lunacy and appoint surgeon and Harvard Law School graduate John Ordronaux the first commissioner. One of Ordronaux's first acts would be to revise the lunacy statutes by tightening up and clarifying how someone could be committed. The new version would pass in 1874. Prior to that, an apothecary could sign a certificate of lunacy, and a clergyman could approve the certificate in lieu of a Judge. Now doctors had to be graduates of "some incorporated medical college" and have been practicing medicine for a minimum of three years. Additionally, their certificates could only be approved by a judge in a court of record.

Nothing more appears about Sister Mary's life in the public record until her death in 1900. She was living alone in a tenement in Brooklyn at the time, and working at St. Vincent's Hospital in Manhattan. She continued to wear a habit and call herself Sister Mary Stanislaus, a Sister of Charity. So, still eccentric. She was much beloved in her building, however, and the children who lived there were accustomed to playing in her apartment at night, perhaps while their parents were out working. On February 3, at 10 p.m., a child reached out and grabbed a tablecloth in an attempt to break a fall. A kerosene lamp on the table started to fall towards the floor along with the child. Sister Mary jumped up and grabbed the lamp, which exploded in her hands. In seconds she was completely covered in flames. The child escaped harm, and Sister Mary died the next morning. She didn't seem to have any old friends or family in her life. Next to almost every section on her death certificate for details about who she was, like the name of her mother or father or how long she'd been living in New York, the coroner wrote *unknown, unknown, unknown.* She was seventy years old.

SUICIDE, MURDER, AND ACCIDENTAL DEATHS
ON THE RISE IN THE LUNATIC ASYLUM

◆

NOTHING CHANGED IN the aftermath of Sister Mary's trials. Everyone at the Asylum, and the commissioners and the public, slowly became accustomed to inaction following a terrible event or disclosure. Visitors, like the people who volunteered for the newly established State Charities Aid Association, a group which was formed to address abuses in the management of the poor, continued to be taken to Hall 3, and they wrote about their investigations, more or less. The superintendents repeatedly drew attention to the same problems, year in and year out, and the commissioners dutifully read their reports. Then coffins were ordered, bodies were piled into them, and everyone turned away as the ferries bound for the potter's field on Hart Island pulled away. The sun would set, the doors would be locked. Doing nothing was how it was going to be.

In the fall of 1873 an economic panic erupted in America and Europe, leading to what would be called the Great Depression, until the one in the 1930s out-greated it and caused most people to forget the other one had ever happened. Although the number of inmates continued to grow in all the institutions that year, there wasn't a dramatic surge. The first hint that an already inhumane situation could still get worse is the fact that the Department of Public Charities and Correction did not issue an annual report for 1872 (which would have been prepared as the Depression took hold). They didn't produce a report the following year either, or the year after that. The Commissioners were either too busy addressing what must have been an increasingly abysmal state of affairs, or they didn't want anyone to know just how bad it was.

Information about those years must be gleaned from later reports and documents, like a letter from Commissioner John Ordronaux, who wrote the President of the Board of Commissioners about the starving inmates of the Lunatic Asylum. Insufficient food, which had always been an issue, was becoming a crisis. "Their only hope of recovery lies in rebuilding the foundations upon which all mental power depends." You must find a way, he implored them. They need "generous nourishment, long and regularly administered." Ordronaux acknowledged the predicament. "I am well aware of the financial limitations under which the commissioners have been placed." And then he made a simple suggestion. All the funds the board received were within its discretion to apply—take money earmarked for something else and put it towards food.

A lack of food was not the commissioners' only problem, however. Up to six women were being locked up in cells meant for one. Building commenced, and by 1875 there were five new pavilions to house the overflow. Three more were completed the following year. But as fast as they could build pavilions, the city committed women to fill them. "This army of wretched inheritors of the worst of all miseries of earth," French wrote, "steadily increases from year to year."

When Dr. Ralph Parsons left to take over the management of the King's County Asylum in Flatbush in 1877, and Dr. William W. Strew took his place, French saw a possibility for change. It wasn't so much that Parsons was doing a bad job; in many ways his hands were tied. But Parsons had managed the Asylum for twelve years. Perhaps a fresh set of eyes were needed. Strew had made a good impression on French, who wrote that his "professional reputation and kindly bearing give promise of all that the poor inmates need and desire." Maybe Dr. Strew would succeed where others had failed.

Strew's initial annual report was full of first-year energy and optimism.

He listed each building and pavilion and outlined precisely how over-crowded they were. If they were going to provide adequate housing, he calculated, they'd need seven more pavilions. In his section about the use of restraints, he agreed with their British colleagues that mechanical re-straints should not be used, but until we have a "sufficiently large and ef-fective corps of attendants" (and about that he complained that they had no fixed standards about proper qualifications), a "reasonable amount of restraint" will continue to be necessary. About their corps of attendants, he applauded the establishment of a Training School for Nurses on the Island, but condemned what they were being paid. "Is it not a mistaken economy to compensate a nurse below what is paid to servants doing housework in private families?"

Strew also drew attention to problems not often mentioned in the an-nual reports. It was known for instance, that a Mary Leinster was both sui-cidal and homicidal and yet nothing was said about this in the certificates of insanity that accompanied her when she was committed. Five days later she was found hanging from a steam pipe. People were not following the proper procedure for commitment.

Under Strew's management, improvements began to take place. The pond in front of the Lodge, which contributed to the unsanitary condi-tions, was filled in and planted with forest trees. New heating pipes were installed in the main building. The bathrooms and water closets got new floors, and renovation began on the older, dilapidated pavilions. In his own 1878–79 annual report, French would finally be able to happily note that he no longer had a makeshift chapel in the hall, but a carpeted chapel room, with a chancel, altar, and lectern, a full set of altar linens, a chest for his books, and a small carpeted vestry room on the side. During services, the chapel became a much-needed refuge for his congregants.

The next year Strew would preside over a promising experiment involv-ing the impact of music. They found that the careful selection of music had a positive effect on the more violent inmates, who "became docile, and shed tears," while previously uncommunicative or combative patients would smile and talk. Like some sort of miracle drug, music seemed to do precisely what they needed it to do. Heart rates were lowered for patients whose pulses were too high, and quickened for patients whose pulse rates were feeble. These outcomes have been reconfirmed today in experiments on responses to music.

Still, there was never enough money. Soon after Strew took over, Josephine Shaw Lowell and Theodore Roosevelt (the father of the twenty-sixth president) sent a letter to the mayor about the budget for the Department of Public Charities and Correction. Lowell was a thirty-three-year-old Civil War widow who'd come from a wealthy and socially progressive family (her brother, Col. Robert Gould Shaw, was the white officer in charge of the black Civil War unit featured in the movie *Glory*). Lowell was also the first female board member of the New York State Board of Charities, and Roosevelt was a fellow board member. They were writing to the city to appeal to them to not only give the full amount the commissioners had asked for the asylums, but even more. Lowell knew all too well what life was like for the inmates of a city institution. She'd been a volunteer for the State Charities Aid Association (SCAA) since 1872, where she regularly inspected institutions and wrote reports, the same tasks she would undertake for the State Board of Charities.

Her capacity for understanding and compassion for the poor in general, however, was not yet fully developed. Like many of her time—and many today—Lowell was a strict proponent of the idea of worthy and unworthy poor. Worthy poor = widows and orphans who were looking for work, the insane, or people who were either too sick, wounded, crippled, or very old. Unworthy poor = everyone else. If you were able-bodied, your poverty could only be the result of a moral failing. You were a drunk, perhaps, or lazy. Other factors like the Depression, or social issues such as fewer opportunities due to race and gender (or, say, being Irish) were not considered. The only way to make you un-poor would be to fix your moral failure.

For Josephine Shaw Lowell that meant packing these "worthless men and women" off to workhouses. Like an Ebenezer Scrooge come to life,

in an 1876 report for the SCAA on "Adult Able-Bodied Paupers," Lowell
called for pulling the able-bodied, whom she called "vicious and idle,"
from "the jails and poor-houses of the State," and committing them, "until
reformed, to district work-houses, there to be kept at hard labor, and educated morally and mentally." The approach may have sounded good on
paper, but workhouses were not very different from jails and poorhouses;
they combined the worst of both, and in practice they never provided the
education Lowell had in mind.

The week before Christmas, Lowell would have another opportunity to
voice her business-like approach to the pauper problem. A six-month-old
baby girl was found frozen to death in the arms of her mother, Julia Deems.
They had been kicked out of their home by Mr. Deems, who was a drunk.
The *New-York Tribune* ran an editorial titled "A Dead Child," which held
the passersby who ignored Julia's pleas for help responsible. A number of
people wrote in to protest. The drunken father was responsible. The city,
which gave licenses to establishments on every corner, thereby relentlessly
tempting men to drink, was responsible. The fact that professional beggars take to the streets with drugged babies (to keep them quiet) was another point to consider. Well-meaning Christians can't give to everyone
who asks and they can't investigate every person for fraud. Besides, there
was also the chance that the money would be used for drink and not to
warm the child. These arguments are not entirely without merit, and are
still made today.

Josephine Shaw Lowell wrote to express another enduring rationale.
"Every woman sitting by the wayside with a baby, who reaps a rich harvest
from the passers by, is a temptation to other women to take to begging as
a profession." Anyone who gives them money only ensures "that the poor
little shivering things will be thrust out the next night also." Since begging
was against the law, Lowell reasoned, the police, who should have arrested
Julia Deems, were responsible. If the police would only do their job, every
one would be sorted out properly—"the really poor would be relieved and
the impostors punished."

No one was more appalled by her response than Rebecca Harding Davis, who was known for writing about social problems of the day. She described Lowell's analysis as "cold-blooded logic" and "narrow and unjust." Were "the rich all honest in purpose and clean in hands when they set about earning a living?" Meanwhile "Julia Deems's child freezes on her breast, while Christian women brush past her and leave her to the police."

It wasn't that Lowell was without compassion, or that she and others hadn't made valid points. The problem was Lowell still believed that if everyone played by the rules the system would work. She had never found herself at the mercy of the police and the courts and the various institutions she championed, and had never experienced first hand how badly they managed to sort out the poor and where they should be sent.

But it was compassion that moved Lowell and Roosevelt to meet with the Board of Apportionment in the mayor's office to discuss increasing the amount of money earmarked for the Department of Public Charities and Correction for the next year, 1878. Unfortunately, like most of the city departments that year, the amount allotted was less than the year before.

For the next two years, the Asylum was thrown into an ever-expanding kaleidoscope of horrors as all the worst-case scenarios they'd been repeatedly warned about came to pass, one after another.

On the morning of May 4, 1878, after finishing her job scrubbing the floors of the Asylum, a sixty-year-old inmate named Anne Hannahan went to the drug clerk to ask for her "rations." Hannahan was what they called a "rounder," a person who was repeatedly committed to the Workhouse or Penitentiary. She'd recently been transferred to the Asylum when she started acting funny, and the rations she was requesting turned out to be a pint of ale.

Alcohol was used medicinally in the nineteenth century. It was prescribed for a number of ailments, such as pneumonia or tuberculosis. In one month at the Asylum, "six barrels of ale, fifty-seven gallons of whiskey, and four gallons of wine" were administered. Even though everyone suspected that Hannahan's intemperate habits were the source of her strange behavior, the daily pint had been prescribed for its therapeutic value as a stimulant. When no one was looking, Hannahan reached up and grabbed a sixteen-ounce bottle of chloroform.

She and her friend Mary Jane Bracken, a forty-five-year-old Workhouse rounder (who'd been confined to the Asylum for epilepsy), took the ale and the chloroform and went up to the fourth-floor bathroom to have a party. When they ran into yet another former Workhouse inmate, Julia Hagan, they invited her to join them. They mixed the ale and chloroform together and downed their cocktails.

They all agreed the drink was horrible, but that didn't stop them from doing their best to finish their glasses. Afterwards Hannahan returned the chloroform bottle to the drug clerk and complained that he'd given her poison. She and Bracken were later discovered wandering the halls in a stupor, and Hagan was found in her room completely unconscious.

The doctors tried everything in their limited array of treatments to restore them. They rubbed the women, and gave them both brandy internally and via hypodermic injections, believing that the brandy could resuscitate them. The doctors also administered electricity, another nineteenth-century medicinal cure. Electric currents would have passed through the women's bodies either via a belt or a harness, or through other appliances. It wasn't generally used on poison victims, but they were running out of options. Hagan died the next day, Bracken the day after. Hannahan, the host and the instigator, survived.

The next month, Bridget Carroll escaped from Pavilion E. She was considered one of the quieter inmates, and had never shown any suicidal tendencies, so they were surprised when her body was found in the river the next day.

In July, Catherine Cavanagh went missing from Pavilion K. Like Carroll, she had never expressed any desire to end her life, but her body was pulled from the river as well.

They found Annie Boyle hanging by her neck in her room on November 23. She'd rolled up a sheet and threw it over a steam pipe that ran through her room.

In spite of all this, and ninety other deaths, Strew's tone in the annual report for that year was upbeat. The main building of the Asylum finally had a proper entrance. Instead of entering through the dank, poorly lighted basement, everyone now climbed up a set of "magnificent and elaborate double stone steps" to a proper sitting room where a huge floor to ceiling bay window had been installed, bathing the room in sunshine and air.

Early the next year, a thirty-one year old named Emily Graham died two days after returning home from the Asylum. Graham had been in and out of the Asylum since the previous October, often ending up in Pavilion G, which Josephine Shaw Lowell would visit later that year and describe as "one of the most painful" places in the Asylum. Graham's doctor was sent for and he reported that her remains were filthy, covered in sores, and emaciated.

A physician on Blackwell's had sounded the first alarm five days before on March 21. "Her body is very much emaciated; she has a bed-sore on right side and two others forming. . . . She has numerous ulcers in various stages of healing . . . a number of scratches on her upper extremities. . . . She has nits on her head. She lies abed in a helpless condition with her legs flexed and drawn over her abdomen. She is unable to straighten them and it cannot be done by force."

Her husband had returned from work at sea to find his previously hardy wife starved, apparently beaten, and afraid of her attendants. He got her out of there at once, but it was too late. On March 26, she was dead. The *New York Times* reporter who saw the body described it as "extremely emaciated" and "covered with putrid sores."

In spite of the condition of her remains, the coroner concluded that Graham died of natural causes, which were chronic inflammation of the membrane of the brain. Although the doctor her husband called in had already been quoted in the papers as saying, "I must express the opinion that her condition indicated at least carelessness and neglect on the part of her attendants," the coroner found that her treatment had been thoroughly humane, and the "charges of carelessness and neglect brought against the Institution are not sustained."

Prior to 1918, when the Office of the Chief Medical Examiner was established, corruption in the coroner's office in New York City was, if not widespread, not unusual. It was possible to buy a favorable ruling at an inquest. Perhaps that's why Josephine Shaw Lowell conducted her own investigation. Although reporters were told that doctors had ordered strong nourishment and three ounces of whiskey a day for Graham, Lowell was unable to find any record that a special diet had ever been prescribed. Without making any definitive accusations, Lowell's report on her findings hinted at the improper use of restraints. Muscles atrophy and contract when someone doesn't move, and it was inconceivable that the Workhouse help who were caring for the Asylum patients would have regularly straightened and massaged Graham's legs to avoid this condition—had a doctor even given that order. Instead, it was more likely she was bound and left largely unattended. Lowell also complained that the coroner's jury never visited Pavilion G, nor did they talk to the nurses who had care of Graham, or her doctor who was young and inexperienced in general and had no background dealing with the insane.

Lowell tried to bring attention to other dangers she'd discovered. More than once she complained to Strew about the burnt matches she found on the floor of the attic in the Lodge during her visits, and still more fire hazards in the cellar. Her efforts did not prevent the fire that broke out in the cellar of the Lodge in May. Given that everyone had to wait for Engine Company No. 39 and Hook and Ladder Company No. 13 to arrive *by boat,* it was miraculous that no one died and damage to the structure was minimal.

In the beginning of his 1879–1880 annual report, Rev. French wrote about "the onward flow of misery." The flow that year included Ellen Welsh, who choked on her food and died on June 5, 1879. It was such a banal death it passed without notice.

The next few incidents that year were so sensational they made the local papers. A pregnant inmate named Emma Morrison had been put in a straitjacket and thrown into solitary on September 11, where she subsequently gave birth. Alone. In a straitjacket. Amelia Doyle died on

September 28 after eating arsenic that was left in the hall by an attendant named Maggie Moedler. Hoping to entice rats, Moedler had mixed butter and sugar into the arsenic, which she then put into a pudding tray and placed inside a pail in the hall. Amelia, who was likely starving, mistook the concoction for actual pudding and helped herself.

Strew suspended Moedler at once. He couldn't actually fire her; the final decision for all hiring and firing came from the Commissioners of Public Charities and Correction. Moedler went over Strew's head and challenged the suspension, insisting on being reinstated. A few months later Josephine Shaw Lowell added her voice to the chorus calling for Asylum managers to be put in charge of hiring and firing, not the politically appointed commissioners. As "long as the Commissioners of Public Charities and Correction are appointed as agents for the distribution of political patronage, no permanent and effective improvement can be made."

But the power to control all the hiring and firing for what would eventually become over twenty-five institutions on five islands—besides Blackwell's, there were facilities on Randalls, Wards, and Hart Islands, and Manhattan—all carrying a combined annual budget of two and a quarter million by the end of the nineteenth century, would not be given up without a battle: imagine three men controlling the operations and employment for the present-day penal institutions, city hospitals, and the Departments of Human Resources and Social Services. The commissioners would remain in charge for many years to come.

Caroline Weill died of starvation on October 10, although Weill's doctor, assistant physician Leonard Pitkin, would immediately claim that this was a fake report put out by Maggie Moedler, who held a grudge against them for suspending her.

By now stories about Asylum abuses were regular features in all the papers. The commissioners of the Department of Public Charities and Correction met on October 27 to discuss the mounting backlash and Strew was directed to start an investigation. The commissioners also asked their Board of Consulting Physicians and Surgeons to conduct their own review.

A week later Strew met with the board to give his report. No one had known Emma Morrison was pregnant, he told them. The assistant physician who'd examined her upon admission had been unable to make a complete examination due to her unruliness. The nurse who was forced to give her regular baths due to her "filthy habits" didn't pick up any sign of her condition either. When Emma complained of abdominal pains they thought it was because she regularly ate grass. Even if they had known she was pregnant it wouldn't have substantially changed how she was treated. Morrison was so violent that putting her in restraints as often as they did was unavoidable. The camisole also helped "protect her from constant nakedness" and kept her from eating her bedsheets and clothing.

The board censured both Strew and the assistant physician for not discovering Morrison's pregnancy, but they deemed the use of restraints in her case an act of humanity and not abuse. They also determined that Caroline Weill did not die of starvation, but had died of an intestinal hemorrhage, confirming the claim that this was a story spread by the bitter nurse. But they rebuked Strew and his assistants for not promptly examining Doyle for arsenic poisoning. Their assessment of the treatment overall at Blackwell's, however, was the most withering. The frequency of the use of restraints, and the brutality of the nurses and attendants, who routinely terrorized the patients with the threat of the crib or straitjacket, could only be addressed by removing Strew, who was clearly unable to manage his own staff.

The commissioners hoped to avoid any unpleasantness by inviting Strew to resign, but Strew refused to slink away quietly, and instead threatened legal action. The commissioners responded by eliminating his position altogether. The next day Dr. Alexander E. Macdonald, who oversaw the men's asylum on Wards Island, showed up to temporarily take charge of the Asylum on Blackwell's.

Strew turned to his attorney, John D. Townsend (the same attorney who represented Sister Mary Stanislaus), for advice. Townsend suggested asking the commissioners to send him the grounds for his dismissal and to give him a chance to explain. The commissioners simply repeated that his position had been abolished, and added that they'd been contemplating relieving him of his duties for some time, due to his inability to enforce discipline.

Strew never took them to court. In 1881, he would run for a seat in the New York State Assembly against Theodore Roosevelt, the one who would go on to become the twenty-sixth president of the United States. Strew lost.

Josephine Shaw Lowell was eventually convinced that "the only radical and effective change which would permanently do away with all the evils that now abound in this institution, would be the removal of the insane entirely from the care of the Department of Public Charities and Correction, and the creation of a separate board to take charge of them. . . . A department which has prisons and alms-houses under its control can never be brought to give adequate care to the insane." Lowell thought a State Board of Lunacy should oversee all the asylums now under the care of both the city and the state.

One week after Strew was removed from duty, Rev. French was in professional hot water as well. He'd made a comment to a reporter about the sorry state of the Almshouse and his Church superiors and the Commissioners of Public Charities and Correction were not pleased. On November 28, 1879, the Committee of Direction of the New York Protestant Episcopal City Mission Society ordered French to write a letter of explanation and apology "in regard to a recent publication relating to the management on Blackwell's Island & that such letter be submitted by the superintendent to the Comm. of Direction & the Commissioner of Charities." French was also told that if he ever did something like this again he'd lose his position.

The spectacular deaths at the Asylum continued.

At 8 p.m. on January 23, 1880, the night nurse Mary Stevens reported for work at the Retreat. The Retreat was a three-story, dark-gray stone building, which sat closer to the Workhouse than it did to the Asylum (it was originally built as a workshop for the Workhouse). Life in the Retreat was often as dangerous as the Lodge, in part because Lodge inmates were moved there when the Lodge got too crowded. The Retreat and the Lodge also shared some of the worst design elements. All the rooms in the Retreat were in the center of the building, which meant they were without windows looking outside or any kind of true ventilation.

Mary Stevens was the only nurse on duty for the entire building, overseeing 157 patients with the help of three women from the Workhouse, one for each floor. Given the crimes that sent most women to the Workhouse, that meant the patients were being guarded either by a thief, an alcoholic, a prostitute, or some combination of the three (which is not to say that thieves, alcoholics, and prostitutes are incapable of compassion, or that they were any worse than some of the nurses appointed by the commissioners).

Stevens and the Workhouse women were expected to periodically walk the halls and peer into the small openings in the doors of each cell to check on the patients locked within. It was also their responsibility to be on the lookout for fires.

Early that morning, at five o'clock, nurse Stevens was jolted by a loud pounding coming from one of the cells. She ran and unlocked the door and found Maria Ottmer, a thirty-eight-year-old German immigrant suffering from dementia, on the floor. Her roommate Lizzie Christ was crouched over her, pounding her head with a wood pail they used as a chamber pot. A third inmate who'd been locked in the room with them was cowering as far away as she could, but in that small space that meant the furthest she could get away from the attacker was ten feet. The nurse ran for help.

A few years before, a system of telegraphic communication had been installed between the Lodge, the Retreat, the Workhouse, and the main building. Stevens frantically telegraphed for help. She likely also rang the gongs that were previously the main method of summoning assistance. When Dr. Leonard Pitkin arrived an hour later Ottmer was still conscious. Despite repeated requests from Stevens, Pitkin refused to have Maria moved to the hospital. Instead, he bandaged her head and left. Ottmer slipped into a coma and was dead by half past seven.

Nurse Stevens was not one of the cruel nurses the patients had learned to fear. Only the month before, she'd written in the Asylum record book of her concerns for the women in her care. "In Retreat Three there are three patients on one side of the room and three on the other. I can't see how they can stand it so close." And only three weeks before she died, when Maria had been too sick and weak to defend herself against her roommates who beat her and dragged her from her bed, Stevens tried to get her transferred to another ward. Maria was kept where she was. After that, Stevens pointed out Maria's swollen feet to an attending physician who did nothing.

Maria Ottmer was no angel. In her stronger and healthier days she was known for destructive behavior and for annoying her fellow patients. She was in the Retreat, the second worst place in the Asylum, because she'd tried to burn the pavilion where she was previously housed to the ground. Somehow she managed to extract from a stove live coals, which she then threw across the floor. Since the pavilions were little more than wooden shanties that were falling apart, and the men of the fire department were a river ride away, she could have killed them all.

Someone had made sure she paid for her stunt. Two weeks before she died her husband visited her and found her in the hospital with a contusion over her right eye. No one would tell him how it happened.

In the month leading up to her death, the record book for the Retreat had several entries concerning Ottmer. December 21: she was described as "considerably emaciated," with several bruises, and "very filthy in her habits." December 27: "Maria Ottmer received a severe beating. . . . Her eyes are much swollen and discolored and there are several scratches on her forehead." Another entry indicated that while she was gravely debilitated due to diarrhea she was never transferred to the hospital.

An inquest into her death was conducted from February 3 to March 15, 1880. The jury deliberated for three hours and came back with the following verdict: "We find that the Assistant Physicians are not sufficiently experienced for the discharge of their duties; their pay is not sufficient to secure competent men. We also find that the pay of the nurses is insufficient to secure competent persons. Maria Ottmer in our opinion should have been treated at the Hospital instead of at the Retreat, and we censure Dr. Pitkin for failing to transfer her to the Hospital when repeatedly called upon to do so by the nurse."

About the overall management of the Asylum, they came to the same conclusions as Josephine Shaw Lowell: "We find a lack of proper system and general irresponsibility. In our opinion the Commissioners in charge of our Asylums and Hospitals should be men qualified by education and training for the position, and should be kept separate from the government of penal institutions. There should be proper accommodation for the patients confined at our Asylums, and we would request the Mayor and Commonalty of the City of New-York to take proper measures for a radical reformation of our Asylums for the Insane."

To call the assistant physicians "inexperienced" was an understatement. Dr. Leonard F. Pitkin was only nineteen years old and an undergraduate when he was first appointed as an assistant physician in 1877, a practice which was not uncommon. He'd only just graduated the year before Ottmer died. The night that she died, all the lives of the inmates in the Retreat were in the hands of a twenty-one-year-old. Pitkin was not fired, but he did leave the Asylum later that year.

The only person dismissed was the night nurse, Mary Stevens. Dr. Alexander E. Macdonald, who'd recently been put in temporary charge of the Asylum, decided that gross negligence on Stevens's part had killed Maria Ottmer. The way Macdonald saw it, Stevens "found the patients quarreling and instead of separating them she locked them in and ran away." He couldn't actually fire her himself. He had to make a complaint to the commissioners who in turn took his advice and removed her. But Stevens had had no good options. She walked in on a large, mentally unstable woman in the process of trying to bash in the head of another. She couldn't separate them herself. If she had left the door unlocked she would have endangered others. The real problems, among many problems she was not responsible for, included the fact that she was alone except for convicts, and when help finally came it was no better than no help at all.

Years later the Asylum would switch to papier-mâché chamber pots "as a precaution against the use of the room vessel for a weapon."

A little over a month after Ottmer's murder, Julia Ablowich and other patients were sitting around a stove in Pavilion G when Julia's dress caught fire. Josephine Shaw Lowell's report calling Pavilion G "one of the most painful" in the Asylum had included a section about the stoves. Lowell specifically noted that they had no guards around them and what a danger that was. This was how Maria Ottmer had been able to draw coals from the fire and fling them to the floor. Lowell's warning did not come soon enough to save Julia. Before anyone could put out the flames she was horribly burned from her feet to her waist. She lived on one more day. Julia was twenty-seven years old when she died, and she'd been on inmate of the Asylum since she was nineteen.

Afterwards, the coroner recommended keeping the stoves unlit until they were properly "caged." But that meant that until they were, the Pavilions had no heating.

Two years earlier Judge John Sedgwick refused to believe that life in the Asylum could be as bad as Sister Mary's lawyer John Townsend had testified, and that was when Townsend had only mentioned the possibility of beatings and the sighting of a single rat. Sister Mary turned out to be one of the lucky ones.

On May 25, 1880, a State Committee on Insanity was appointed to investigate abuses in the management of insane asylums. They were instructed to explore all asylums in the state. At the top of their list was the institution that had prompted the investigation in the first place, the infamous New York City Lunatic Asylum on Blackwell's Island.

LUNACY INVESTIGATION

December 1880

Metropolitan Hotel, New York City

———————◆———————

THE DEPARTMENT OF Public Charities and Correction was always in over its head. In 1880, the year of the Senate investigation, 8.4 percent of the entire population of New York City had come under its care (although perhaps a little less, given that some of the inmates were repeats). Other states were escalating the crisis, the commissioners complained, by sending their blind, lunatic, and infirm poor to New York in order to "rid themselves of pauper burdens." The Asylum superintendent was forced to concede that due to the overwhelming numbers, "proper classification is unattainable at present," essentially making the whole concept of moral treatment an impossible dream. While they would not have relished defending themselves against the perception that they were the source of the problem, perhaps like Moses Ranney all those years ago, the managers of the Asylum hoped that all this attention would finally lead to change.

The special committee was made up of three senators: William B. Woodin, a Republican and the chairman of the committee; Charles A. Fowler, a Democrat; and Edmund L. Pitts, a Republican. They met for the first time to hear from witnesses on Wednesday, December 1, in Parlor No. 125 at the Metropolitan Hotel at Broadway and Prince Street. Issues that had been raised many times before were revisited, like overcrowding, the use of restraints, a shortage of attendants, and the fact that the commissioners were not medical men and the superintendents didn't have backgrounds in caring for the insane. They heard from doctors, nurses, experts in the study of insanity, commissioners, superintendents, ex-superintendents, clergy, and members of the State Board of Charities. But they didn't elicit testimony from a single patient.

The first witness sworn in was Dr. Edward C. Spitzka, a twenty-eight-year-old alienist (the nineteenth-century term for psychologists and psychiatrists) whose specialty was "diseases of the mental and nervous system" and who, according to later testimony from Dr. Alexander Macdonald, had been rejected by no less than five asylums where he'd applied for a position. Spitzka, a member of the American Neurological Society (who would go on to become their president), would disprove this claim.

Perhaps the real reason for Macdonald's animosity towards Spitzka was that the year before, the American Neurological Society had submitted a petition to the state legislature outlining asylum abuses, and that part of the problem was that superintendents and their assistants were not keeping up with the times. They are "not versed in the new anatomy and physiology of the nervous system," and "are not believed to be skilled in the modern methods of diagnosis and post-mortem examination." Macdonald would later tell a reporter that Spitzka and the Society were enemies of all "superintendents of insane asylums they could not control."

According to Robert Whitaker in his book *Mad in America*, neurologists like Edward Spitzka "prided themselves on being men of hard science" and saw the "asylum doctors as a pathetic lot—old, old-fashioned, and hopelessly influenced by their Christian beliefs." The Society's petition maintained that doctors in the asylums wasted time writing "useless histories of cases" and "talking by the hour with friends of patients."

Spitzka did a very clever thing. When asked to state what he knew about abuses in the management of asylums he simply read from one of the hospital books that was used to record accidents. His selection of brief but striking entries revealed more of a war zone than a refuge, making it very clear how someone like Maria Ottmer could end up murdered by a patient wielding a chamber pot:

> August 21, Rose McLaughlin, received yesterday from Hall 5, made a furious attack on the nurses last evening and it became necessary to place her in restraint; has received several severe bruises on her left shoulder and arm, and large discolored patches and several scratches on her right shoulder.
>
> September 25, Charlotte Marsh was attacked suddenly and without provocation this morning by Mary Sullivan; received a blow on the head inflicting a severe wound.
>
> December 21, Maria Ottmer, considerably emaciated; is very filthy in her habits; there are several discolored spots on the body which were present the day before.
>
> December 27, Maria Ottmer received a severe beating from Sarah Way; her eyes are much swollen and discolored and there are several scratches on her forehead.
>
> September 1, Anna McKenna was attacked and beaten by Ann Scott, receiving several severe bruises on her body.
>
> October 8, Mary Stuart became violent this morning about 5:30; attacked the nurse with a heavy wooden pail.
>
> October 12, while Mary Stuart was in a paroxysm of excitement, a few days ago, she struck Emma Limburger with a pail.
>
> October 13, Augusta Klink, became excited yesterday evening and fell forward to the floor, dragging with her the bench to which she had been strapped by a belt owing to her destructiveness; she struck her head, inflicting a very severe bruise, which has an extensive swelling and discoloration about her eye.

When he got to the entry noting that Maria Ottmer had not been transferred to the hospital after having been attacked, he read a selection of other sick or injured patients who were never sent to the hospital:

September 27, Johanna Hanser has a high, fever, her pulse being very rapid; complained of pains and vomited; she was not transferred to the hospital until the next day, as she was violent, and the physician hoped she would recover.

October 1, Adelaide Hahn has a high fever; she was not transferred to the hospital, as she might injure other patients. The witness added that this patient was kept continually in restraint.

October 3, Clara Krans, a patient who had been struck in the Retreat on September 28, and had not been transferred to the hospital then, very much exhausted and seems to be growing weaker. She has several bruises, probably caused by falling from her bed; was transferred to hospital next day, and then died.

A doctor who'd been present at the inquest into Maria Ottmer's death testified that Dr. Leonard Pitkin's testimony (the doctor who refused to move Maria to the hospital) "would have disgraced a first-class horse medical student in his utter ignorance of the system." Everything about the management of asylums had to be overhauled, he continued, but in particular the practice of hiring inexperienced young men like Pitkin, then turning them "loose in insane asylums, apparently under the presumption that the insane, of all classes of invalids, require less medical care."

That it was as bad as the doctor said was later confirmed by Josephine Shaw Lowell. A young physician from Blackwell's had confided to her, "We go there to learn. Of course we make horrible mistakes. . . . And when we learn all we want to, we resign and another greenhorn is put in." In two years, she told the committee, there have been eighteen different physicians. Eighteen rounds of horrible mistakes.

Much of the Committee's focus was on restraints. Physician after physician protested about their excessive usage. Dr. William J. Morton, a professor at the University of Vermont, described seeing a particularly agitated patient in a crib. The man was "in the frenzy of melancholia, and his beating about the cage, it was a very horrible spectacle. . . . I thought at the time it would be a great mercy if they would tip it on end, and give him a chance to stand up, or give him a chance to sit up, but this forcing him to lie on his hands and feet, it seems to me a very cruel process."

Dr. Thomas M. Franklin, who had taken over the Asylum from Alexander E. Macdonald, was asked about what kind of restraints were in use.

"We employ the camisole mostly; we employ wristlets to a small extent, and we own one or two muffs, and we use that much-abused institution, the crib or protected bed, of which we own four and of which I wish we owned more."

Senator Woodin had to make sure he heard correctly. "You would employ more if you had them?"

"Yes, sir." He was having one built right now for a new patient, as a matter of fact, and he was hurrying "its completion for her use" out of a "sense of duty." Besides, cribs looked worse than they actually were.

"Did you ever try to take a night's rest in one of them, doctor?" Woodin asked.

"No, sir."

"Wouldn't that be about as good a way to determine whether it is altogether comfortable or not; with the lid fastened down I mean?"

"I think not, sir. . . . It prevents no motion except that of sitting up," Franklin responded.

Woodin wouldn't let him off the hook. Trying spending a night in one, "with the lid locked down."

The Reverend William Glenney French made his first appearance at the inquiry on Monday, December 6. "You hold a communication in your hand," Woodin began. It was an urgent telegram French had received the night before from his superior, the Rev. Curtis T. Woodruff. "Will you allow me to take the communication?" Woodin asked. French stepped forward. "Of course I am very glad to further personally any examination into lunatic asylums. . . . But this stops me at present." The Senators read the telegram and conferred. "Well, we will allow you to halt here for the time and that is all." But he was expected back there the very next morning at 10 a.m. One more thing, the committee asked, how might we find Rev. Woodruff? We want to have a word with him as well.

William W. Strew, the former superintendent, was sworn in a little later. Strew immediately defended his tenure at Blackwell's. He claimed his ouster was all political theatre. There "had been so much said in the papers about the complaints about the institution," Commissioner Brennan had told him, "that they felt there must be something done; somebody must be sacrificed to political necessity."

"Did they use that language?" Woodin asked.

"Yes, sir; it was a necessity. If I did not resign their heads would have to come off." Given what so many others had said about how politics influenced appointments, Strew's claim had the ring of truth. Further, he argued that his difficulty in maintaining discipline was due in part to the commissioners themselves. He would suspend an incompetent worker only to have the commissioners return the worker to duty. "It creates a spirit of exultation first, and insubordination. . . . They regard it as of little account, because they have got a power behind the throne that they can go to—the Commissioners."

Perhaps Strew was no worse than any of the previous superintendents. Maybe in one respect a little better. The senator's questioning revealed that it was Strew who instituted the practice of keeping track of the use of restraints in a separate log book. "When I went there I found they were in the habit of using restraint indiscriminately. . . . One of the first and worst abuses that my attention was called to was its use by the attendants unknown to the physicians, and by the physicians to gratify the attendants unknown to the Superintendent. If a patient was in any way troublesome and they required to be with her and watch her they found it much more convenient to strap her in a chair or put her under restraint so that they could go and attend to their own business or do something else. Consequently there was too much restraint used, altogether." The log book introduced at least some measure of transparency.

The news of French's eleventh-hour communication from his superior had made the rounds and the next morning Parlor No. 125 was as crowded as Sister Mary's courtroom had been. Everyone leaned left and right, in an effort to catch a better view when French's supervisor, the Reverend Curtis T. Woodruff, superintendent of the New-York Protestant Episcopal City Mission Society, who'd received his own eleventh-hour communication—a subpoena—was sworn in. The *New York Times* wrote that Woodruff, whom they described as "short and stout," and with a "florid complexion," took the stand "with ill-concealed diffidence."

The exchange between Woodruff and the senators was lengthy and heated, and the following is an edited version of what took place (as are all the questions and answers between the other witnesses and the senators in this chapter).

With Woodruff's telegram in his hand, Senator Fowler got right to the point. "You state here to Mr. French, 'you have no business to testify before that Committee (meaning this Committee) at all.' On what do you base that statement?"

"On the ground, sir, that he is not supposed to know any thing about what has transpired on the Island at all; he is forbidden by the rules of the society to do any thing, except attend to his own spiritual matters."

"You state in this letter that if he testifies he does it at the risk of losing his position."

"Yes, sir."

"Do you mean to say that this society which is a society in my own church would dismiss a faithful servant for telling the truth under compulsion?"

"No, sir, I do not mean to say such a thing as that at all."

"Are you conscious of the fact that the subpoena of this committee compels his attendance under pain of imprisonment?"

"Yes, sir, I am."

"Well, what do you mean by that when you say that if he testifies he does it at the risk of losing his position?"

"The fact, sir, that he can testify at all disqualifies him according to the rules of the society from being an employee of the society."

"If while he were holding religious service there an attendant should in cold blood murder a patient, would he be discharged because he saw it and was compelled to testify to the fact?"

"No, sir, I suppose not."

But Woodruff's reluctance was not about the rules of the Society, it soon became clear, it was about avoiding displeasing the Commissioners of the Department of Public Charities and Correction, who could kick them off the Island at any time and not allow any from their Society to return. French had almost been banned from the Island by the commissioners when he went to the papers with "charges of various kinds against the Commissioners of Charities and Correction as to the internal affairs of the Asylums," Woodruff testified. The commissioners thought it was "unfair; he is there by the courtesy of the board, and it is unfair for a man who has the freedom of the Island, the right to go in and out of the wards freely as the spiritual adviser, to take advantage of his position and bring to the public things that he may hear; little abuses, or large abuses, whatever they may be. They think it is unfair and unjust, and I think you can but feel it, it is so, sir; if a minister should come into your family to advise your patients would you think it right for him to go down into your kitchen to look at the food you ate, and interview your servants?"

"And you think these are analogous cases?"

"I think they are, sir."

"He is there discharging a duty . . . to a class of unfortunates who cannot speak for themselves and you regard that as analogous to a meddlesome Paul Pry coming into a private family?"

"He is there to spiritually advise the patients and nothing more; his duty stops there."

"Then you think if a person occupying the position Mr. French does, as a witness of abuses it is his duty to keep it from the public?"

"His duty is to communicate it to me and I have from time to time communicated with them [the Commissioners of Charities and Correction]. . . . My object was simply to come before you gentlemen and appeal to you as gentlemen and Christian gentlemen not to interfere with the work of the Society by requiring one of our missionaries to come before a board and testify to abuses or things he may have seen while in the discharge of his spiritual duties."

"I think it is the opinion of this Committee that if your Society tolerates abuses there and conceals them from the public the quicker you are got off the Island the better it is for those poor unfortunates there."

Over Woodruff's protests, Senator Fowler read Woodruff's letter to French aloud.

From the office of the New York Protestant Episcopal City Mission Society, at 306 Mulberry Street. New York, Dec. 6, 1880.

It is now just half past nine o'clock and you are not summoned to appear before ten A. M.

You had no right to go away without seeing me first; you have no business to testify before that committee at all, for you are not supposed to know anything at all in regard to the abuses, if any exist, in the asylum. You testify at the risk of losing your position; read what is said on page twelve of the by-laws, which I send you by bearer. Your simple duty is to read your plain instructions and say that you have nothing to testify about the internal affairs of the asylum. That don't [sic] come under your jurisdiction; you are there only to care for the spiritual welfare of the inmates and nothing more. It was very wrong in you not to wait and see me, for we could have talked the matter over and decided what to do. As I said before you will testify at the risk of losing your position, for there is a strong feeling in the board on the subject in regard to what has transpired in time past, and a stronger feeling on the part of the commissioners.

Hoping you will consider these things.

Truly yours,

C. T. WOODRUFF, Superintendent, etc.

"You never attempted to investigate any of these alleged charges of abuses existing?" Fowler asked.

"No, sir, I did not, because it was not my business," Woodruff replied.

"Would you not regard it as a part of your duty to inquire into any grave abuse of twelve or fifteen hundred helpless lunatics?"

"I should not; I am there for a different purpose."

"The church then, or the City Mission Society, cares nothing at all for the temporal wants and physical comfort of these unfortunates, but only looks after their spiritual welfare?"

"That is it, except so far as they do individually, sir; they give refreshments and various little things patients may need, but nothing further. They feel they have no right to say any thing or ask any questions."

"I am a little curious to know what this City Mission Society deems its duty in a case of this sort, and therefore I ask you whether, if Mr. French should see a brutal assistant murder a patient, he would incur the displeasure of this Society if he interfered to protect the lunatic?"

"Well, I do not know; I could not answer such a question as that; you might ask me the same question with reference to a man in the street; if he should stop and look on and see a brawl, he could or not interfere as he saw fit."

"Will he be discharged if we force him to testify?"

"I think not, sir; he will be discharged, if at all, because he has allowed himself to go outside of his regular duty and see these things, and look into these other matters that belong to other people, and not him."

"You had better employ a blind man," Senator Pitts spat out.

"Yes," Senator Fowler added in disgust, "and a man without any bowels of compassion."

Once more Woodin tried to make Woodruff concede the moral imperative. "If he tells the truth and speaks of abuses . . . wouldn't it be right, if he knows the fact of abuses, to state them?"

But Woodruff would not concede. French should have "simply attended to his spiritual duties and nothing more. . . . That is the true course for a Christian minister to take."

And with that, Rev. French, whom the *New York Times* described as a "venerable old man, with kindly lineaments" was recalled. Many years later, in his obituary in the *Churchman*, French would be commended for his actions on this day. "The active and manly part which the single-hearted missionary took in bringing about these reforms is a matter of civic history." They praised how "he did not hesitate to give evidence, both full and free," without mentioning how the Society did everything it could to prevent him.

After eight years on the Island, French had accumulated "some five or six folio manuscript books and four or five quartos" worth of entries about what he'd witnessed, and he had a lot to say. He began with the story of Jane Stevens, a woman around thirty-five years old who'd regularly attended his services. When she didn't show up for a few weeks he went looking for her. He found her outside, sitting at the foot of a tree.

"You have not been to my service for two or three weeks. What is the matter?"

Stevens told him that she'd been transferred from the relatively pleasant Hall 3, where French conducted his services at that time, to one of the much less desirable Pavilions. When she refused to leave the Hall without first collecting her clothes, the nurse got two men who "took her by the shoulders, one on each shoulder, and pushed her out and pushed her along to the stairs," roughing her up so badly she'd been crippled and unable to stand ever since. (The newspapers had reported at the time that she'd been pushed down the stairs. French stopped short of making this assertion.)

A nurse and others later confirmed to French what Jane had told him.

"What subsequently became of this woman, Jane?" senator Pitts asked.

"She was removed to the alms-house and put into the hospital, and died there . . . a little over a year ago," French answered, adding that he "never, from the first to the last, saw any thing in her that indicated insanity, except when she first went in there. She had been disappointed in love, she said, outside, and she did not care whether she lived or died."

"Do you know what occasioned her death?"

French had asked the young physician in charge of the hospital if her death could have been the result of how she'd been treated, and was told "that it could have easily come from it."

When French spoke to a reporter about what happened to Jane Stevens, the commissioners punished him by taking away the special key he'd been given with access to all of the Asylum.

"I would like to say to the honorable committee," French added, "that I have disagreed in principle from the Society and Superintendent in regard to my duty as a Christian and a man."

"That is obvious enough by your keeping this record," Senator Woodin responded, referring to his journals.

French then told them the story of Sister Mary Stanislaus, who he knew well, and how she had been mistreated and locked up in solitary, in a room too dark for him to peer into, all because she had sought help for a fellow patient.

"Do you know the name of the nurse and attendant?"

"I know the name of the nurse; she is dead, sir. I know she was a very cruel woman."

This led to French unburdening himself of one evil it's clear he'd wanted to talk about for some time: the nurses and attendants. Some "were compassionate, considerate to the patients, and apparently did everything in their power to make them comfortable; and I have known others that I should judge from their treatment of the patients had no higher idea of their duty than a herdsman would have with a company or herd of beasts. . . . Many of them have not humanity enough to be a nurse, and some of them have not intelligence enough; some of them have not education enough; and perhaps what is more important than all in my estimation, they have not tact, tact and sympathy," nor, he added, "patience."

"Neither the commissioners nor the doctors, the chief nor the assistants could discover, unless it were by accident, many things that have been done, and probably many things that are done and will be done," French continued. "The physicians generally make one visitation during the day, unless called specially to go the rounds; after that time the patients are in the hands of the nurses entirely."

"You think the fault of the system is that it is infected with politics?"

"I think that almost every evil that has been connected with the institution would be remedied in time, and a very speedy time, if there were no appointments made of any but intelligent, humane, conscientious people—sympathizing people."

French had never spoken to the commissioners, or anyone at the asylum, about the abuses. Not only did he feel he could "not remedy it," he thought he "might produce more trouble in the remedy." But he did tell Rev. Woodruff. "I have told him of cases, these and others, and told him at the same time that I felt as if it was a duty to bring those things before the Commissioners. . . . He usually put the matter aside by saying that they did not care [to] interfere with such things." French testified for a while longer, and then he was asked to review his notes and come back another day.

Commissioner Townsend Cox wasted no time in giving his opinion about French when he was sworn in a little later.

"I thought Mr. French seemed to be more of a meddling old woman than a missionary, from certain actions of his, and it seemed as if he was more interested in giving items to reporters than he was in any good that might come to the inmates of the institution; he seemed to be more inclined to try to get up a sensation in the newspapers than to do any good."

"Did you ever think to inquire into them, to see whether they were true or not?"

"I don't remember whether we did or not; most likely we did."

"Don't you think now that was a matter of sufficient importance to have called for some action, investigation or inquiry on your part?"

"We no doubt did investigate, but I cannot remember in this particular case."

French was quick to defend himself when he returned the following day, December 9. "If in this I act the roll [sic] of the meddlesome old woman . . . I accept the term as of the highest honor. I have never communicated with any reporter, save one—and it was a misfortune which came near my downfall. He did not record me correctly . . . I came very near being dismissed from the island."

French had many years to consider what he said soon after.

"Place a nurse or attendant in charge of a large hall containing over seventy patients, such nurse appointed by political influence, without regard to education, moral character, training for the special work, humanity, good temper and conscience, and we can easily see what might be done. . . . Nurses chosen without respect to their fitness in any respect for the place, and shut up in a hall like those halls of the asylum, we can imagine any thing almost to be done with impunity."

"Go on then?"

"The buildings are such that anything might be done which an ignorant, cruel or passionate nurse or official might be prompted to do. . . . The nurse has full control and . . . any deed could be committed, and no testimony of the patient would be believed against the word of the nurse. The patient is supposed, being in a lunatic asylum, to be incapable of giving testimony against an official."

"What do you mean by that?"

"Well, sir, if a patient were to make complaint to the principal officer, the nurse would be brought in, and by her explanations of the matter could set aside any thing that the patient could say in her own behalf."

"And no further notice taken of it?"

"No further notice taken of it."

French gave an alarming example of brutality ignored. "Within the last two weeks a young lady—a nurse—of her own accord told me that the reason why her mother, also a nurse and a very kind-hearted lady, left the island was her indignation at the cruelty of a fellow nurse who held a patient of filthy habits from disease, in the water of the bath until her face was livid. The daughter told me that both her mother and the fellow nurse were sent before the Commissioners, but both were continued on in office, but her mother found herself so worried in the place that she resigned and is now engaged in private nursing. I would add that the nurse who did that is at present a nurse in the institution."

"Now have you any objection to giving the names of those who were witnesses to it?"

French gave them names, Mary Williams and her mother, but the two women were never called. French also testified about the practice of bathing many women in the same bath water, a fact that he'd heard from so many sources he had absolutely no doubt it was true. "The water was put into the bath and . . . one after the other, as many as could be bathed at a time, passed through it unchanged."

In spite of the fact that this practice had been reported many times, and had come up in investigations before, the senators didn't believe him. How could any one patient know how many people had been in the same bath water before and after unless she remained in the bathroom the entire time? It's not clear if Dr. Parsons was in the room when French addressed bathing at the Asylum, but he would have been able to confirm that not changing the water between bathers was standard operating procedure. He'd written about it in the Department of Public Charities and Correction's 1867 annual report.

The Senate committee continued to hear testimony through to the following year and a report was issued on April 5, 1882. It was presented without making a single recommendation for improving the management of the insane.

The following April the *American Journal of Insanity* printed a response.

This document consists of about one thousand pages. Persons were examined at various periods down to the close of the legislative session of 1881, and the committee was continued with a view of further inquiry and authorized to report at the legislative session of 1882. At that session the committee submitted the testimony and reported that they had no recommendations to make.

After running over the "evidence" we can well understand why the committee had nothing to recommend. In the whole mass of testimony there is not a new idea in regard to legal provisions for admission, discharge, organization, management or internal administration of asylums. . . . Most of the "witnesses" . . . are persons who have figured before the public for some years past in the role of lunacy reformers in various associations, periodicals and pamphlets which they have given wide circulation, and their "testimony" is merely a re-hash of all this. The "testimony" of several consisted very largely in quotations from the reports and writings of Dr. Gray, Dr. Macdonald and other members of the Association of Superintendents, and of assertions and allegations, but nothing really rising above the grade of misrepresentation, cavil and quibble.

French's testimony was not mentioned.

Meanwhile the Asylum population kept growing. In their 1881 annual report, the Department of Public Charities and Correction commissioners lamented the "constantly menacing increase of the insane." The use of restraints also continued unabated, only now whenever patients in camisoles left the Asylum, they were covered with shawls to hide them.

In 1886, the position of General Superintendent of the New York City Asylums for the Insane was created, and Alexander E. Macdonald, who had testified before the Senate committee in 1880 (and was called "backward" by Dr. Edward Spitzka), was appointed as the first General Superintendent. The institutions he was now responsible for were:

Pavilion for the Insane at Bellevue Hospital
The New York City Lunatic Asylum on Blackwell's Island
The New York City Asylum for the Insane on Wards Island
The Idiot Asylum on Randalls Island
The Branch Asylums on Wards, Hart, and Randalls Island
The farm on Long Island

There were moments in Macdonald's 1880 testimony where he admitted things were truly horrendous at the asylums, and that change was needed. He had addressed their absurd and inhumane budget, which was already low when the per capita allowance per patient had been 37 cents, but they were now "clothing, feeding, treating, housing and warming our patients for the sum of twenty-four cents a day each." To keep costs that low, inmates were fed crappier and crappier food, and less of it.

But he never reached the level of frankness that is found in his first report as General Superintendent in 1886. The promotion seemed to have filled him with purpose. Or perhaps he resented having to answer to the state and now that he wasn't being interrogated he felt free to tell the truth.

Because he now confirmed what both French and Strew had testified six years earlier, that at the hand of the attendants, "instances of neglect, even of violence, are of far too frequent occurrence." And, on the few occasions when attendants were found guilty of deliberate cruelty or of being drunk on the job, they were allowed to resign and then were rehired soon after. Macdonald also confessed that for the commissioners, getting costs down was paramount, and "the nobler office of curing them becomes of secondary importance. . . . To be sure some of them will die, but so much the better for the tax-payers!"

French's annual reports were equally dark. The year Macdonald was made the first General Superintendent, French wrote, "Blackwell's Island, as a whole, is the cesspool of New York City."

Women were still being housed in the Lodge even though the building had been condemned. Repeatedly. Death rates at the Asylum, which were already considered deplorable, continued to rise. Ninety-eight people died in the Asylum in 1880. In 1887, a year after Macdonald was appointed, the number was up to 173. Perhaps this was because since 1880 the "constantly menacing increase of the insane" had grown 28 percent.

As these terrible numbers continued to soar, a twenty-three-year-old novice journalist named Elizabeth Cochran was offered an assignment of a lifetime. Her editor asked her if she'd be willing to get herself committed to the Lunatic Asylum in order to write under cover about the alleged abuses. She couldn't resist. The articles she wrote for the *New York World* came out soon afterwards in a book titled, *Ten Days in a Mad-House*. Ten days was all she could withstand. There were cruel nurses in her account, too, and stories so over the top her report reads like a script for a horror movie.

NELLIE BLY

Ten Days in a Mad-House

September 1887

———◆———

T HE ASSIGNMENT HAD come from John Cockerill, the managing editor of the *New York World*. In his obituary it was said, "He was a fighter if there was fighting to be done." And he knew how to choose a worthy soldier. The investigation would make Cochran famous, but she'd become known by her pen name, Nellie Bly, given to her by a previous editor who took the name from a Stephen Foster song, although he got the spelling wrong (it's Nelly). Did Bly know at the time that Foster had died a pauper in the charity ward at Bellevue Hospital, managed by the same commissioners who ran Blackwell's Island?

Bly was not the first to write such an exposé. Julius Chambers, who attended Sister Mary's trial and shared the same lawyer, did something similar for the *New-York Tribune* fifteen years earlier in 1872, when he was twenty-one years old and had voluntarily committed himself to the comparatively pleasant Bloomingdale Asylum (although not so nice for everyone there, he would uncover). But Chambers was not the journalist Bly was, and he got some of his facts wrong. He described Sister Mary as "a spinster, possessed of a large fortune" when she was a nun without a penny. His exposé did lead to the release of several sane people who'd been improperly committed, however, according to Chambers, and likely contributed to the tightening up of the lunacy laws in 1874.

As soon as Bly stepped onto the boat that would take her to the Island she could see it was bad. She almost collapsed from the breath of an attendant who reeked of whiskey, before she made her way to a filthy cabin guarded by two women. "They were coarse, massive women, and expectorated tobacco juice about on the floor in a manner more skillful than charming." When they got to the Island she asked where she was. "Blackwell's Island," she was told, "an insane place, where you'll never get out of."

Her account tells the stories of fellow inmates, like Tillie Mayard, who was perfectly rational at first, although frail. And Mrs. Louise Schanz, who appeared to have ended up on Blackwell's because she couldn't speak English. "Confined most probably for life behind asylum bars, without even being told in her language the why and wherefore. Compare this with a criminal, who is given every chance to prove his innocence. . . . Mrs. Schanz begged in German to know where she was, and pleaded for liberty," but no one listened.

During the admission process Nellie's doctor did little more than check her height, weight, and coloring, and he paid more attention to the nurse than to Bly.

From there her account confirms every horrible story inmates and visitors to the Asylum had been telling for decades. Her first meal was served in the basement and consisted of a slice of bread, five prunes, and a cup of tea. The bread was immediately stolen by the woman sitting across from her.

Her first bath sounds like the precursor to waterboarding. "The water was ice-cold, and I again began to protest. . . . My teeth chattered and my limbs were goose-fleshed and blue with cold. Suddenly I got, one after the other, three buckets of water over my head—ice-cold water, too—into my eyes, my ears, my nose and my mouth. I think I experienced some of the sensations of a drowning person as they dragged me, gasping, shivering and quaking, from the tub. For once I did look insane." Patients with "the most dangerous eruptions all over their faces" dried themselves on the same towels Bly was expected to use. She used her underskirt instead.

When Tillie Mayard complained about the rough treatment during her own initial bath, the attendant Miss Grupe answered, "Shut up, or you'll get it worse." Grupe then warned Bly, who'd asked for a nightgown, to not "expect any kindness here, for you won't get it."

That night Bly found a spider in her bread. "I tried the oatmeal and molasses, but it was wretched, and so I endeavored, but without much show of success, to choke down the tea."

In her first walk outside, Bly witnessed a wagon procession, the device used to safely take the women from the Lodge on walks, and the one which the creator thought would be viewed as a happy parade. Bly saw "a long cable rope fastened to wide leather belts, and these belts locked around the waists of fifty-two women," who passed her by "staggering, pulling, jerking, screeching, crying, singing, preaching, swearing . . . like lost souls marching into a furnace in Hades."

She confirmed what the Senators refused to believe about the bathing practices on the Island. "On bathing day the tub is filled with water," Bly wrote, "and the patients are washed, one after the other, without a change of water. This is done until the water is really thick, and then it is allowed to run out and the tub is refilled without being washed."

One day, Emmet C. Dent, the newly appointed medical superintendent of the Asylum, came through the sitting room and stopped to talk to some of the patients. At thirty years old, Dent was a relatively young man. He'd recently placed an advertisement for junior medical staff to help him. The ad stipulated that there would be no pay, but board, lodging, and washing. "Duties are principally medical, and no better opportunity can be had for the study of insanity."

Bly encouraged her fellow patients to tell Dent "how they were suffering from the cold and insufficiency of clothing," but they declined. The nurses would beat them if they did, they told her.

It wasn't long before Tillie Mayard's health began to fail. During an examination, Bly asked Dent and his assistant to look after Tillie instead, but they paid no attention to her pleas. When Tillie herself got up and asked for help they ignored her, too. "The nurses came and dragged her back to the bench, and after the doctors left they said, 'After awhile, when you see that the doctors will not notice you, you will quit running up to them.'"

On her next visit with Dent, Bly tried to talk to him about everything she'd witnessed. "I told of the state of the food, the treatment of the nurses and their refusal to give more clothing, the condition of Miss Mayard, and the nurses telling us, because the asylum was a public institution we could not expect even kindness." Dent did in fact check in on Tillie afterwards, but "he caught her roughly between the eyebrows or thereabouts, and pinched until her face was crimson from the rush of blood to the head, and her senses returned. All day afterward she suffered from terrible headache, and from that on she grew worse."

Bly finally found a kind soul when she appealed to the assistant superintendent of the Asylum, Dr. Frank H. Ingram, who at twenty-seven was only a few years older than Bly. There was perhaps a hint of attraction between the two. In her account she described him as the "flirty young doctor." When Bly told him the inmates were freezing, Ingram ordered the attendant Miss Grady to give the patients more clothing. Miss Grady promptly threatened Bly that if she made a practice of complaining to the doctor, she'd regret it.

On another occasion Bly confided to Ingram about her fear of patients dying in a fire after they'd all been locked in their rooms for the night. "The nurses are expected to open the doors," he responded. Bly immediately countered, "But you know positively that they would not wait to do that . . . and these women would burn to death." He asked her what they should do about it, and Bly noted with irony that he was seeking advice from "me, the proclaimed insane girl." But Dr. Ingram was the one person who was not convinced that patient Nellie Bly was insane. He felt her case didn't fit "any of the recognized types of insanity," according to a later issue of the *Medico-Legal Journal*.

The torments continued. Bly described how Miss Grady and other attendants started teasing a patient.

They kept up this until the simple creature began to yell and cry. . . .
After they had gotten all the amusement out of her they wanted and she
was crying, they began to scold and tell her to keep quiet. She grew more
hysterical every moment until they pounced upon her and slapped her
face and knocked her head in a lively fashion. This made the poor creature cry the more, and so they choked her. Yes, actually choked her. Then
they dragged her out to the closet, and I heard her terrified cries hush into
smothered ones. After several hours' absence she returned to the sitting-
room, and I plainly saw the marks of their fingers on her throat for the
entire day.

This punishment seemed to awaken their desire to administer more.
They returned to the sitting-room and caught hold of an old gray-haired
woman whom I have heard addressed both as Mrs. Grady and Mrs.
O'Keefe. She was insane, and she talked almost continually to herself and
to those near her. She never spoke very loud, and at the time I speak of
was sitting harmlessly chattering to herself. They grabbed her . . . by her
gray hair and dragged her shrieking and pleading from the room. She
was also taken to the closet, and her cries grew lower and lower, and then
ceased.

It was just as French had warned seven years earlier, "nurses chosen
without respect to their fitness in any respect for the place, and shut up in
a hall like those halls of the asylum, we can imagine any thing almost to be
done with impunity . . . and no testimony of the patient would be believed
against the word of the nurse."

Patient after patient related similar stories to the one French had told
seven years earlier about the nurses who'd held an inmate's head under
water. Bly reported on a Mrs. Cotter who was sent to the Retreat after running towards a man she had mistaken for her husband. "For crying the
nurses beat me with a broom-handle and jumped on me, injuring me internally. . . . Then they tied my hands and feet, and, throwing a sheet over
my head, twisted it tightly around my throat, so I could not scream, and

thus put me in a bathtub filled with cold water. They held me under until I gave up every hope and became senseless."

Bridget McGuinness, who experienced the same mistreatment, talked about what the nurses did to make sure they got away with it. They "would always keep a quiet patient stationed at the window to tell them when any of the doctors were approaching. It was hopeless to complain to the doctors, for they always said it was the imagination of our diseased brains, and besides we would get another beating for telling. They would hold patients under the water and threaten to leave them to die there if they did not promise not to tell the doctors. We would all promise, because we knew the doctors would not help us, and we would do anything to escape the punishment."

Even for death there were no repercussions. After breaking a window Bridget was transferred to the Lodge. "While I was there a pretty young girl was brought in. She had been sick, and she fought against being put in that dirty place. One night the nurses took her and, after beating her, they held her naked in a cold bath, then they threw her on her bed. When morning came the girl was dead. The doctors said she died of convulsions, and that was all that was done about it." One hundred seventy-three women died in the Asylum in 1886. How many of those deaths came about through similarly suspicious circumstances and were ignored?

Bly talked about being locked in a room with six other women and her fears of a danger that actually had occurred more than once in the past. "Two of them seemed never to sleep, but spent the night in raving. One would get out of her bed and creep around the room searching for some one she wanted to kill. I could not help but think how easy it would be for her to attack any of the other patients confined with her." Dr. Ingram, her protector, had her moved to a quieter ward, which also happened to be away from the bullying Miss Grady.

Bly described how they were made to sit all day on benches without a book or anything to distract or fill up their time, something French had witnessed and tried to address. It was probably the least sensational section of Bly's account, and yet the quiet cruelty is in some ways the most ghastly.

I was never so tired as I grew sitting on those benches. Several of the patients would sit on one foot or sideways to make a change, but they were always reproved and told to sit up straight. If they talked they were scolded and told to shut up; if they wanted to walk around in order to take the stiffness out of them, they were told to sit down and be still. What, excepting torture, would produce insanity quicker than this treatment? Here is a class of women sent to be cured. I would like the expert physicians who are condemning me for my action, which has proven their ability, to take a perfectly sane and healthy woman, shut her up and make her sit from 6 A.M. until 8 P.M. on straight-back benches, do not allow her to talk or move during these hours, give her no reading and let her know nothing of the world or its doings, give her bad food and harsh treatment, and see how long it will take to make her insane. Two months would make her a mental and physical wreck.

Bly never mentioned the use of restraints, but she did write later that the inmates were "continually dosed with chloral to keep them quiet."

Towards the end of her report Bly wrote, "The insane asylum on Blackwell's Island is a human rat-trap. It is easy to get in, but once there it is impossible to get out. I had intended to have myself committed to the violent wards, the Lodge and Retreat," but when she learned from inmates how perilous those places were, "I decided not to risk my health."

Her *New York World* articles caused a sensation, and were reprinted all over the country. Soon after, Bly appeared before a grand jury and was questioned by Assistant District Attorney Vernon M. Davis. The jurors and Bly then left for what they thought would be a surprise visit to the Island. But the commissioners had been alerted about the visit, they learned. When the jurors walked into the kitchen on Blackwell's they found it clean and brimming with food. The halls were also spotless, and the inmates clothed and presentable.

General Superintendent Alexander Macdonald, who was in charge of all the New York asylums, would argue that in the few days that Blackwell's allegedly had to prepare for the visit, "it would have been impossible to revolutionize the management of a public Institution containing 1,600 inmates and to reconstruct its arrangement and rehabilitate its dependents." But they certainly had time to sufficiently clean up the place and the inmates, stock up on food, and then threaten the women to not say or do anything to indicate that this was not business as usual.

Medical Superintendent Dent conceded that "the food was not what it should be," but they bought what they could with their pitiful budget. Insufficient funds were also the reason they couldn't attract the best doctors and attendants to the Island. But when he said he had no way of knowing how many women were bathed in the same water, or if the nurses were cruel, there is no other way to put this: he knew he wasn't telling the truth. These facts had come out many times before, including in their own annual reports.

To Bly he said, "I am glad you did this now, and had I known your purpose, I would have aided you. We have no means of learning the way things are going except to do as you did. Since your story was published I found a nurse at the Retreat who had watches set for our approach, just as you had stated. She was dismissed." But what about the nurses who were doing whatever it was their colleague was making sure the doctors wouldn't witness?

Medical Superintendent Dent would continue to manage the Asylum, and he would go on to become a big proponent of, ironically, hydrotherapy. In 1902 he wrote proudly of the new treatment he used on an eighteen-year-old working girl. She'd been suffering from fear and delusions, along with auditory and visual hallucinations, and she was brought to Dent in a highly agitated state. First they gave her a large enema. Then they irrigated her stomach with water and force fed her with a stomach tube. After that they wrapped her in warm, wet sheets, which they covered with blankets, putting an ice pack on her head and a hot water bottle at her feet. They left her like that for three hours. This treatment was continued regularly for a week, then followed up with other various water treatments before they discharged her four months later, fully cured, Dent claimed. Hydrotherapy was popular for a time, minus the stomach irrigation and force feeding that Dent prescribed.

Dent complained that they shouldn't be faulted for pronouncing Nellie Bly insane when she did everything she could to make them believe she was. What reason did they have for not accepting that her behavior was genuine? It was a valid point, except according to Bly, as soon as she was admitted, "I made no attempt to keep up the assumed role of insanity. I talked and acted just as I do in ordinary life."

Bly feared that the grand jury would not accept her account "after they saw everything different from what it had been while I was there. Yet they did, and their report to the court advises all the changes made that I had proposed." Which included hiring female physicians. Drs. Alice E. Wakefield and Augusta A. Steadman were employed the very next year, although like their male counterparts, they didn't stay long. But other female doctors would take their place. One of them, Dr. Louise G. Rabinovitch, would come back in 1894 to testify (along with Alexander Macdonald) at yet another Senate hearing about abuses in insane asylums.

"I have one consolation for my work," Bly wrote, "on the strength of my story the committee of appropriation provides $1,000,000 more than was ever before given, for the benefit of the insane."

The Board of Estimate made their own visit to the Island in December 1887, however, and ultimately an $850,072 increase was approved (nearly a 57 percent addition over the previous year). The Department of Public Charities and Correction had already asked for a higher apportionment before Bly's report ever came out, but it's thanks to Bly that they got as much as they did.

The additional money didn't result in a substantial increase of quality of life for most of the inmates. The amount spent on the women per day was only raised from 23 cents to 31 cents. There also wasn't enough for significant building. A hothouse to grow flowers for the wards was erected, and building commenced on a nice home for the attendants. This was done with the idea that it would help them attract a better class of women. Given that the attendants were previously housed in the same buildings as the inmates, and under at least somewhat similar conditions, that must have been true. More attendants were subsequently hired and at a higher pay scale.

But the Lodge was finally and truly condemned, and walls were moved in the Retreat so that the rooms were no longer in the center of the building but in the surrounding corridors. Now each room had a window, along with heating and ventilation. In addition, a new fire escape was planned, work on a bathhouse was begun, and money was put aside the next year for a new pavilion.

Where they were previously issued thin shawls for winter, and that was it, the women now got ulster coats (an overcoat with a cape, fashionable for the day) which were made by the patients themselves from blankets. Perhaps the most surprising use of the additional money was the purchase the following year of twenty-five canaries bought for the wards along with "many bright table covers and other decorations." But the tiny songbirds were a compassionate and perceptive purchase. Scientists have since confirmed that the sounds of certain birds have a restorative effect and can relieve stress.

The "flirty" Dr. Ingram left his position at Blackwell's later that year to enter private practice. From time to time he would testify as an expert witness on insanity. (He was present at Thomas Edison's laboratory when two calves were electrocuted to demonstrate that the electric chair was a more humane method of execution than hanging. "The calf was cut on the foreward and on the spine behind the forehead," a *New York Times* reporter wrote, "and sponge-covered plates, moistened in a solution of sulphate of zinc, were fastened in place.")

Bly and Ingram remained friends after her release, and there were always rumors that their relationship had blossomed into something more. After making her famous seventy-two-day trip around the world in 1890 (beating the fictional expedition of Jules Verne's 1873 novel *Around the*

World in Eighty Days by a week), she stopped in Ingram's hometown in Indiana. A local reporter asked if there was any truth to the rumor that they were engaged. Bly fueled the fires when she would only say that she knew him "intimately." Ingram felt compelled to write the paper from New York to deny the rumor, but added that he was nonetheless an ardent admirer of Nellie Bly. The paper accepted the denial, but the wording (and Bly's response) seemed to indicate that there had been a romance at one time; it just hadn't led to something more serious. Three years later Ingram would die unexpectedly of a heart attack. He was only thirty-three years old.

Bly would look back at her time on Blackwell's Island and call it the "ten longest days of my life." Assured that something was being done, most people moved on. Bly had a more realistic outlook. Of the women she left behind she wrote, "I left them in their living grave." In spite of her excellent work, the abuses and the inhumane conditions continued. French would note the improvements in his annual report that year, but conclude, "Duty to God, and duty to our fellow man, and especially to that portion of our race, which for her helplessness, ought to secure from men mercy and justice, but does not."

A few months after Bly's report came out another husband, Ernest Schmidt, visited his wife in the Asylum and found her bruised and emaciated. The nurses said her injuries were due to falls and fights with her fellow patients, but his wife Emelia strongly denied their claims. Schmidt turned to lawyer August P. Wagener, who the year before had successfully won the release of thirty-eight people from the insane asylum on Ward's Island. It took Wagener two months, but on February 29 Schmidt was finally able to bring his wife home to their two small rooms in the rear house of 160 East Third Street. In a brief interview with a reporter, Emelia said she was afraid to name the people who abused her, but things had been all right for a few weeks after she'd been moved out of Ward Six. "I was well taken care of and happy, but then a new nurse came, and—and—and—I am happy I am home." Emelia died the next day. The esteemed coroner

Michael J. B. Messemer performed the autopsy, attributing her death to "Exhaustion from endo- and pericarditis, pleurisy and nephritis."

"Nowadays that would be classified as something like 'Systemic septic complications of endocarditis,'" according to forensic pathologist Dr. Jonathan Hayes, "which is an infection of the heart valves or inner lining of the heart."

Messemer also said her brain showed "unmistakable traces of insanity." "There would be no 'unmistakable signs of insanity' in the patient's brain," according to Andrew Scull, a professor at the University of California at San Diego. "Except for cases like Alzheimer's disease, there aren't any visible even with today's much improved techniques and microscopy, and certainly nothing would have been visible then." Even at the time they acknowledged how little they knew. In his books Scull quotes Dr. David Ferrier, who spoke before a London committee on a hospital for the insane in 1889. "Much has been written on the symptomatology and classification of the various forms of insanity; but I think we really know nothing whatever with regard to the physical conditions underlying those manifestations. Until we are able to correlate mental disorders with their physical substrata, and this we are very far from being able to do, we cannot be said to possess any real knowledge on the subject."

As always, the commissioners and the Asylum managers were found blameless in Emelia's death. The women on the Island would have to wait until the state once again felt compelled to intervene and finally take a step for which many had been crying for decades.

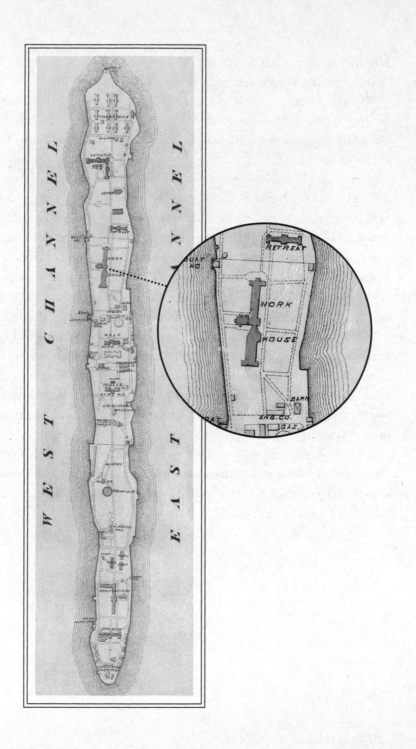

❧ II ❧

THE WORKHOUSE

———◆———

A PENAL INSTITUTION FOR PEOPLE CONVICTED
OF MINOR CRIMES, OPENED ON BLACKWELL'S ISLAND
IN 1852, FOR SENTENCES GENERALLY
TEN DAYS AND UNDER

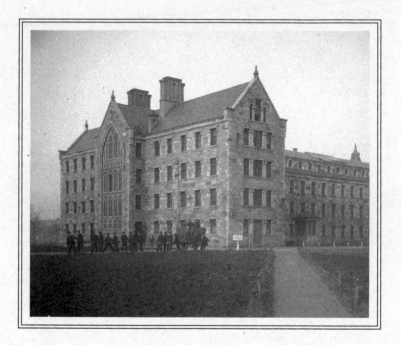

NEW YORK CITY AND THE UNWORTHY POOR

TEN YEARS AFTER the first patients were transferred to the Lunatic Asylum, the Common Council turned its attention to another group it intended to isolate on Blackwell's Island: people convicted of minor crimes and the criminally lazy, otherwise known as the "unworthy poor." An act to establish the Workhouse on Blackwell's Island passed on April 11, 1849, and within two months people were being committed to a institution that didn't yet exist. The police justices were less than enthusiastic about sentencing convicts there at first. However, a clause in the act allowed the commissioners to pull together a group of able-bodied men from the Almshouse and give them this choice: commit yourself to the Workhouse or leave. The newly christened convicts were immediately assigned the task of building the future prison. It was like ordering them to dig their own graves. (At least two men would die during construction.) When Rev. French arrived on the Island years later he would describe the two wings of the Workhouse as "exactly in the shape of huge coffins; fit receptacles of a multitude dead in soul."

It was the prison you see in old movies. A friend of a later warden would describe it as a "strangely dramatic and terrible building." Made of the same gray Fordham gneiss as the other institutions on the Island, it had a few gothic touches and a pervasive air of gloom. The design has been attributed to James Renwick Jr., who was the supervising architect for the Department of Public Charities and Correction at the time. Renwick is known for two other gothic structures in New York City: Grace Church at Tenth Street and Broadway, and St. Patrick's Cathedral on Fifth Avenue. Perhaps the ecclesiastical windows above the entrance to each wing, which added an element of beauty to an otherwise austere, foreboding structure, were a contribution of Renwick's.

Once again the commissioners scaled back from an initial design of four wings to two. The final two wings, Renwick would point out in the Department's annual report, could "be constructed at some future period, when the wants of the city may require them." The important consideration was, "there are few, if any, buildings at present in the country which have been constructed with more economy than the Work House."

The male convicts were housed in the south wing, the women in the north, and the two wings came together at a center building which faced the East River and held, among other things, the quarters for the superintendent, chaplain, and various officers, along with a kitchen and a chapel. There were also smaller buildings on either side of the end of each wing, forming an L, that contained additional facilities like dining rooms, workshops, and a laundry.

Each wing was 291 feet long and 50 feet wide and held three tiers of cells on both sides of a great hall that was open from the floor to the ceiling. A keeper (the same as a prison guard) standing at the end of the hall would have a sweeping view of the iron stairways leading up to narrow balconies running along the sides of each tier, and all the cells lining the three floors.

The cells for the men and women were designed a little differently. In the women's wing there were twenty-five cells on both sides of each tier, or 150 total. Each cell was meant to hold four people, and was a little bigger than other cells on the Island: 16 feet long, 8 feet wide, 11 feet high. The men's cells on the first tier were the same, but on the second tier there were fewer but larger cells designed to hold sixteen people. On the third tier, they were larger still and held twenty-four. Unlike some of the buildings at the

Lunatic Asylum, all the cells had windows, except for six "dark" cells—the name for solitary at the time—which were located on the ground floor. There was also a padded cell on the ground floor, generally used for people suffering from delirium tremens.

Municipal leaders still believed in institutionalization and classification, and the restorative value of correctly identifying either the crime or the mental illness, and subsequently installing each inmate in an institution specially designed for their respective classification. But they also understood that they had gotten it wrong so far, and they saw the Workhouse as their best chance to get it right. Although they didn't know it at the time, it would be their last chance, at least on Blackwell's Island. Except for the Smallpox Hospital, which opened in 1856, the Workhouse would be the last major institution erected there.

The Workhouse was envisioned as "intermediate department between the Penitentiary and Almshouse," a place for minor criminals, vagrants, and the able-bodied poor. It would be the institution that would finally achieve just the right balance between punishment, charity, and reform. Small-time criminals didn't really belong in the Penitentiary, and poor people who were still capable of work didn't belong in the Almshouse. With a little bit of creative reshuffling, all the populations of the institutions of Blackwell's Island could finally be put right.

As the work on the buildings progressed, the commissioners gave the order to pull vagrants and the drunk and disorderly inmates from the Penitentiary, and the able-bodied poor from the Almshouse, and transfer them all to the Workhouse. Inmates were classified and separated according to age, sex, and the severity of their crimes. The young, and the first offenders, were to be kept apart from the more habitual, predatory inmates, who would destroy them, thereby avoiding the pitfalls of the Penitentiary, which had become a school for even greater crimes. Over in the Almshouse, only the old and the infirm (the "worthy poor") remained. From now on, people who were out of money and options but still capable of working would no longer be considered appropriate candidates for the

Almshouse. A penal institution was the proper place for their kind, and they were welcome to voluntarily commit themselves to the Workhouse if they were looking for a handout.

The other option, providing relief to the poor in their own homes, was seen as an evil that would discourage them from improving their lot. The only truly effective way to eradicate poverty was to commit the poor to institutions like the Workhouse, where the reasons for their destitution—their supposed moral failings and loathing of hard work—could be cured. How the commissioners expected to accomplish this was made clear in the 1852 annual report, in which the first superintendent of the Workhouse quoted another writer on the subject. "The Work House should be a place of hardships, of ample, though coarse fare; it should be administered with strictness—with severity; it should be as repulsive as is consistent with humanity. . . . It is most unjust, as well as most detrimental to the moral being of the individual, to encourage him in idleness by the gratuitous offer of a better, at least, a sufficient subsistence." Tough love.

Like the Lunatic Asylum, the Workhouse failed virtually from the start. A later warden would call it "an almost complete model of what such an institution should not be." More than any other initiative on Blackwell's Island, the Workhouse embodied the competing aims of the Department of Public Charities and Correction and the City of New York, demonstrating conclusively that dispensing punishment and charity at the same time is a balancing act that is nearly impossible to achieve, even with the best of intentions. And when other needs, like economy, trump everything else, it is impossible.

The Department's first problem was, as always, way too many poor people. Once again the commissioners greatly underestimated the size of the population they intended to serve (and reform). In 1850, 1,182 men were sentenced to the Workhouse (while living in the Almshouse as they worked on building the new institution). By the time Rev. French arrived on Blackwell's Island in the 1870s, 20,000 to 33,000 people were being sent to the Workhouse every year. Even given the fact that a certain percentage of those numbers were "rounders"—the same people being committed repeatedly—the Workhouse soon had the largest and most transitory population on Blackwell's Island. It also became the biggest correctional institution in New York City, and most of the inmates came from the place that had been initially reluctant to sentence people there, police court.

When someone was arrested in New York in the nineteenth century, they were first brought to the station house and then to police court. By 1874 there were five in Manhattan and one in the Bronx. The police justice would then either discharge the prisoner, hold them for trial in one of New York's superior courts (the Court of Special Sessions for serious misdemeanors, or the Court of General Sessions for felonies), or, because the justices had the power to render judgments for ordinance violations and lesser misdemeanors, they'd either fine them or send them to the Workhouse. The Workhouse became *the* "prison-house for commitments by police justices."

Referred to as the "poor men's courts," the six police courts operated like conveyor belts of sorrow. One by one, people would step out of a pen and up to a rail in front of a raised platform called "the bridge," where the arresting officer stood above them, conferring out of earshot with the judge. Because they couldn't hear, many didn't find out they'd been sentenced to prison until they were shoved into a police van and taken to the Twenty-Sixth Street Pier. Given the number of people arrested each year and the fact that the justices not only didn't show up every day but sometimes only worked through the morning, sentences were passed on up to seventy-five or more detainees every session. Prisoners were lucky if they got better than a minute or two of consideration on a busy day.

Corrupt justices would dismiss the few cases of the wealthy and politically connected, or impose a fine or bail which they could easily pay. This left the unconnected poor, who couldn't make bail and were instead sent to the Workhouse (like arrestees today, who are sent to Rikers Island when they can't make bail). Sometimes people were sent to Blackwell's simply because the defendant didn't speak English and packing them off to the Workhouse was easier than finding the interpreter. Years later, the Women's Prison Association would describe how prisoners with influence were let off easy while others would be committed with apparently "no reference either to the prisoner or to the crime, but rather upon the good or bad humor of the justices."

The justice's power to sentence or pardon was tremendous, and lucrative. If bail was set at $500, the accused would have to either pay 10 percent of that amount to a bail bondsman or go to prison. The bondsman would then split the $50 among some combination of the police justice, the lawyer, the arresting officer, clerks, and others. On a good day they could be dividing up $1,000 or more. "The shyster lawyers hand in glove with the clerks and the police attendants," wrote the Charity Organization Society of the City of New York, "wrung from the distracted inmates of the detention pen the last dollar they possessed." (Today the poor are fleeced in additional ways, with an array of court fees, fines, and financial penalties for paying late.)

There was almost no oversight. These were the poor and minor criminals, after all, and few were looking out for them. Things finally got so out of hand that papers like the *New-York Daily Tribune* blasted the system, writing that "no civilized community on earth was ever worse served than New-York has been under the administration of the police courts. . . . They are not merely a reproach to this city, but a virulent poison which has infiltrated the body politic and is steadily spreading corruption."

The police courts were abolished after an investigation in 1894, and replaced with the magistrates court. Justices now had to be attorneys-at-law, appointed by the mayor. (When New York was consolidated, there would be a total of six magistrate courts in Manhattan, two in the Bronx, eight in Brooklyn, three in Queens, and two on Staten Island.) There was some improvement at first, but the abuses slowly resumed. By 1907 the situation was "so notoriously bad" the Charity Organization Society of the City of New York pointed out an article published in *Broadway Magazine* titled "The Farce of Police Court Justice in New York: Magistrates, Lawyers,

Ward Heelers, Professional Bondsmen, Clerks of the Court and Probation Officers Join to Make a Mockery of 'The Supreme Court of the Poor.'" In the article, Franklin Matthews, a night city editor at the *New York Times*, described a heartless system that shook down and imprisoned their most vulnerable citizens (Matthews would go on to become one of the first professors at the Columbia School of Journalism). The Society fought successfully for the appointment of what became the Page Commission, which investigated the courts, leading to the passage of the Inferior Criminal Courts Act in 1910 and further reforms.

MOST OF THE people locked up in the Workhouse had been arrested for intoxication, disorderly conduct, vagrancy, or prostitution. For crimes like intoxication and disorderly conduct, those who could afford to paid a fine and were sent on their way, which again left only the poorest doing time. That time was usually brief. Although occasionally someone might receive a sentence as long as a year, and other sentences could be anywhere from one month to six, the majority of Workhouse sentence were ten days or less. Turnover, therefore, was high. And one particular group was going in and out of the Workhouse more than any other.

Although the female wing of the Workhouse was the last to be completed, by 1857, when the figures by gender began to be supplied regularly, the yearly totals for women were higher than the men's, sometimes a lot higher, such as during the Civil War years. That would continue to be true until 1883, when men finally started edging out the women in numbers. Still, for much of the second half of the nineteenth century it would appear that more women were going to prison for minor crimes than men.

The problem is the yearly totals included rounders, and do not represent the total number of unique individuals sentenced. Workhouse superintendents often said there were more female rounders than men, and many of those commitments could have been the same women being arrested over and over. But the superintendents never supplied enough information to verify their claim, and the figures they did provide came from the inmates themselves. Periodically they asked the men and women, were you ever sentenced here before?

It can only be said that women were sentenced to the Workhouse with greater frequency, and that may have been due to fact that judges were harder on women for the crime that was most likely to get you sent to the Workhouse: disorderly conduct. According to *Abbott's Cyclopedic Digest of all the Decisions of all the Courts of New York From the Earliest Time to the Year 1900*, disorderly conduct referred to "offenses less than felony against the peace or good morals of the community."

In practice, disorderly conduct meant whatever the police and the courts wanted it to mean and that was likely the intention behind the broad wording of the statute. What constituted proper behavior for a woman was narrower than what it was for men, and the law became, in part, a catchall to keep women in line. The 1860 act lists streetwalkers, for instance, but not their customers. An 1888 police justice came right out and declared that for women only, simply being out at night was probable cause. The way he saw it, "no decent, respectable woman would be found in the street without an escort after 10 P.M.," and therefore, he told a Women's Prison Association investigator, "any woman alone in the street after that hour ought to be arrested." Accordingly, at night police would sometimes sweep up women by the dozens. Although some of the women rounded up were undoubtedly prostitutes, the male criminals also out and about after ten were not picked up just for being on the street after dark. When brought to police court, the Women's Prison Association investigator found, the women were immediately sentenced without being given the time to gather their thoughts and speak for themselves, or to produce witnesses.

It's no surprise then that for crimes like disorderly conduct, the conviction rates were higher for women. For example, while 71.5 percent of the people brought to court for disorderly conduct between 1885 and 1895 were men, the average conviction rate was 80.6 percent for women, and only 65.5 percent for men.

In 1893, Reverend Charles H. Parkhurst, who was waging a campaign against prostitution, would say that he didn't care if working girls were thrown out of disorderly houses (houses of prostitution) to "starve or freeze on the streets," as long as they were "starved and frozen" into another way of life. "If Doctor Parkhurst wishes to suppress this great evil," activist Matilda Joslyn Gage shot back, "he should turn his attention to the men. . . . He can have every disorderly house watched, and every man entering it arrested, fined, and his name published. That would put a stop to it speedily."

A committee investigating police corruption in 1895 wrote how "in a number of cases women, who, as keepers of disorderly houses, had paid thousands of dollars for police protection, had become reduced to the verge of starvation, while those who had exacted blackmail from them were living in luxury."

Economics contributed in other ways to the number of women who ended up in the Workhouse. Fewer labor opportunities and lower pay meant that once convicted, women were less able to pay fines to avoid incarceration, so off to the Workhouse they went.

This was a more serious matter than being simply unfair. On Saturday, February 17, 1866, nineteen-year-old Fanny Little was picked up for the two crimes that landed most people in the Workhouse: intoxication and disorderly conduct. Forty-two other people were arrested in New York that day, twenty-five men and sixteen women (the name of one arrestee was gender neutral). Some paid their fines or made bail and went home. But the highest bails imposed that day, $300 or $500, were all for women. Being drunk in public was inexcusable for a woman. One annual report of the Board of Police Justices bluntly stated that "public exhibitions of drunkenness in females indicate a depraved and abandoned condition," while men were sometimes let off the hook because in their case there were often "circumstances to be taken in mitigation of punishment which rarely exist in cases of females."

Fanny, whose bail was set at $500, was ultimately sentenced to five and a half months in the Workhouse. ($500 is not an unusual amount for someone arrested for disorderly conduct today.) If she'd received even a slightly shorter sentence, she might have made it out of there alive.

On July 22, when she was a little less than two weeks short of being released, Fanny got sick. Twelve hours later she was dead, the first casualty of a cholera epidemic. If she'd started showing symptoms earlier, they were ignored, but she had their attention now. "A sensation then commenced, never witnessed in this or any other department," wrote the superintendent of the Workhouse, "each individual appeared perfectly panic-stricken." (A reasonable reaction.) Before it was all over, more people died of cholera on Blackwell's Island than any other area in New York City, perhaps in part because police justices continued to send people there, even though the epidemic didn't end until the last week of September. In total, 360 people died of cholera on Blackwell's Island that year and the Workhouse was hit the hardest. Two hundred four of the inmates who were incarcerated there during the epidemic fell ill, and ninety-seven women and fifty-one men, plus two employees, died.

WORKHOUSE CONVICTS WERE processed similarly to Lunatic Asylum patients. Once sentenced, convicts were taken from the Tombs (the nickname for the city jail) to the docks at the foot of East Twenty-Sixth Street. There they'd board the same Department of Public Charities and Correction steamboat as everyone else bound for Blackwell's Island, except they'd be locked up in the cabin. At the Workhouse, the clerk would enter them into the admission book, noting their crime and sentence, and a few personal details like their occupation and place of birth. The scrubbing, which came next, was the same scene of horror it was at the Lunatic Asylum, with everyone sharing the same bathwater. After their bath, regardless of what they came in wearing, inmates were supplied with clothes made by fellow prisoners, and which, as usual, often fit neither the wearer nor the weather.

The work inmates were assigned would depend on their skills and what was needed at the time in the Workhouse and the other institutions managed by the Department of Public Charities and Correction. Although superintendents were accused of exaggerating just how productive the inmates were—some inmates were so idle for much of their time in the Workhouse they referred to it as a "House of Rest"—life inside the Workhouse usually meant work.

The nature of the work changed over the decades. In the early years they had a cigar shop and a hoop skirt factory (contracted by manufacturers in the city). The Workhouse also had a carpentry shop, tailor shop, shoe shop, sewing room, boathouse, blacksmith shop, barber, stables, and a vegetable garden. The men tended to work outside, on the steamboats, at the quarry or stone shed, in the gardens, stables, and a bake shop, and they did all the building, repairing, and road work. They also commanded the tailor and shoe shops, and the kitchen. The women sewed, knitted, helped in the kitchen, joined the men in the tailor shop, or were assigned to the scrubbing gang who washed down the floors daily. But the women got out of the Workhouse, too. Despite the fact that, according to one superintendent, "a majority of the inmates of the Work House stand very low in the scale of intelligence, and therefore may be considered in the same light to their officers as children to their parents," these were the women the commissioners saw fit to send out to look after helpless patients in the Lunatic Asylum and other institutions on Blackwell's and the other islands. Some made the most of their time outside the Workhouse. They'd be sent to the infants' hospital on Randalls Island in the morning and come back drunk that night, the Women's Prison Association reported in 1888.

Workhouse tasks were often morbid. The annual reports listed every job performed and each item produced, which taken together sometimes foreshadowed the whole tragic arc of so many of their lives. The more imaginative among them must have been haunted by their assignments. A select group of men in the Workhouse were sent to the morgue to receive and prepare the unclaimed dead for dissection, while other inmates were later dispatched to the city's potter's field to bury them. The men would have wrapped the pauper dead in shrouds that came out of the Workhouse sewing room, and placed them in coffins built in the Workhouse carpentry shop.

The production numbers themselves tell a macabre story. One thousand shrouds came out of the sewing room in 1886, and 1,731 adult coffins and 1,186 children's coffins were assembled in the carpentry shop in 1860. The chamber pots which on several occasions became murder weapons in the Lunatic Asylum also came out of the Workhouse carpentry shop. The inmates even made the straitjackets and other restraining devices that most Asylum superintendents claimed to barely use. But someone had to have ordered the 146 restraining jackets, 36 restraining dresses, 145 restraining straps, 24 restraining muffs, 6 restraining belts, 24 restraining gloves, and 30 pairs of wristlets that were produced by Workhouse prisoners in 1879. Given that someone who was a Workhouse inmate one day could the next day become a Lunatic Asylum patient or an unclaimed body in the morgue, a worker could have been building his own coffin or sewing her own straitjacket or shroud.

The mortality rates for the Workhouse were actually comparatively low, and as long as you didn't have the bad luck of being sentenced during the occasional epidemic you had a decent chance of getting out of there alive. (Mortality rates were sometimes kept artificially low; Workhouse inmates who died in other institutions they were transferred to were not always included in the yearly totals.)

As in the Lunatic Asylum, there were times when inmates died shortly after going home. In 1875 Jacob Stockvis, who suffered from an unidentified mental disorder, wandered from his home. The police, not recognizing his disorder, arrested him for drunkenness and disorderly conduct. Then, without any prompting, evidence, or testimony, the police court judge threw in a charge of "collecting a crowd and fighting" and sentenced him to six months in the Workhouse. Stockvis, who was speechless due to his affliction, could say nothing in his defense. Back at the station house, he was badly beaten by a fellow inmate and transferred to the Workhouse without receiving any medical attention.

His family, who looked everywhere for him, finally found him a week later in the Workhouse and brought him home, but it was too late. He died the next night. The jury at the inquest said his death was hastened by a "want of medical aid and proper treatment and nourishment after his arrest and while confined in the station-house of the Nineteenth Precinct, in the Police Court Prison, and in the Workhouse on Blackwell's Island."

The jury criticized the Commissioners of the Department of Public Charities and Correction, noting that "the manner of distributing the prisoners after their arrival in the Workhouse on Blackwell's Island is irrational, and their treatment during their confinement is, in many respects, degrading, and demands thorough investigation and reform." And while they were very careful to say, "we deprecate all attempts to encourage weakness and leniency in the arrest and punishment of vagrants and criminals, as such leniency would increase the audacity and recklessness of a dangerous class of our population," no one had checked Stockvis's injuries. No one made an effort to ascertain his mental condition. No one made sure he was properly fed. Who was the truly dangerous class? The jury recognized this on some level, because all of that said, they added that there "should be a more strict and thorough system of examination and discrimination . . . and more uniform laws relative to the dispensation of justice."

Most people managed to remain alive through their stay in the Workhouse because their sentences were so short they weren't there long enough to be killed by disease or starvation or abuse. If inmates did get sick, they were treated in "hospitals" located at the end of the male and female wings, in the L sections, each with around twenty beds. Ordinary prison cells were also set aside in each wing for sick inmates who didn't require constant supervision, and a cell on either side was used as a dispensary. There was even a cell on the women's side that was used to perform operations.

It was a classification issue. They wanted to keep the prisoners away from the Charity Hospital patients. It was also another example of how they never got classification right. Sick Workhouse inmates deemed too dangerous to be among the innocent poor were relegated to an in-house hospital, while healthy Workhouse inmates were sent to the Lunatic Asylum and other institutions virtually unsupervised.

The standard of care in the Workhouse hospital was unconscionably lower than what patients at Charity Hospital received. Although there was no running water above the second floor, the hospitals were set up on the fourth floors. According to an 1888 Women's Prison Association report describing the hospital on the women's side, the facility was "frightfully over-crowded . . . dirty, the beds infested with vermin." Open and uncovered chamber pots left out for patient use were only "flushed occasionally by a bucket of dirty water." A single nurse was hired to care for all the sick in the hospital, with only prisoners as assistants, who in turn gave out medicine while making frequent mistakes with "not infrequently, serious consequences." (The assistants were often illiterate and couldn't read the directions for medicine they were expected to administer, and some depended on memorization.) Standard medical practices were ignored. Inmates "with contagious eye diseases are placed, side by side, with other patients; the nurse attends to the eye troubles, and immediately goes to another patient."

Disease and contagion weren't the only things the women in the hospital had to fear. "A warrant for the arrest of one of the physicians has been issued within the last few months," the 1888 Women's Prison Association annual report noted, "for an attempted criminal assault on one of the women." The saddest revelation was the fact that women who were suffering from chronic disease were kept in this makeshift hospital after their prison sentence was over. Instead of being transferred to the more humane Charity Hospital, they'd remain in this inferior penal ward until the day they died. It was a life sentence by default, for a minor crime that others had evaded with connections and a small fine.

Reports of the hospital on the men's side are not as revealing, with only occasional mentions of repairs made, like an unsafe ceiling being plastered, or additions like a new operating room which was outfitted in 1892.

Ultimately the successful and vindicating classification that commissioners and reformers hoped for never transpired. Like all the other institutions on the Island, inmates in the Workhouse were not segregated as intended, according to their age or crime. Boys were housed with men, girls with women, and the able-bodied, self-committed poor were put in cells alongside those habitually convicted of actual crimes. Not only did the Workhouse fail to solve the Island's classification problems elsewhere, it exacerbated them. As if anticipating criticism, the commissioners wrote that this was a situation "it is a great deal easier to decry than to find a remedy for."

It's not as if they hadn't been trying to fix the problem almost since the first piece of granite on Blackwell's Island was laid.

REV. WILLIAM R. STOCKING

Superintendent of the Blackwell's Island
Workhouse from 1886 to 1889

———————◆———————

As reverend french made his way around the Island he would have passed by convicts cutting stone, building sea walls, or pulling beets and turnips from the garden. He did not have the same unfettered access to Workhouse inmates that he did with the patients at the Lunatic Asylum. He was not supposed to stop and talk to them. He was only given time and space for one service a month at the Workhouse, and generally only about seventy-five people out of all the inmates, anywhere from 800 to up to 1,500 on any given day, showed. Making even a spiritual dent in such a large and guarded population was going to be difficult.

But French was immediately drawn to the people in the Workhouse. He didn't see them as the borderline idiots the superintendents described, although he did concede at times that perhaps some of them found themselves in the Workhouse due to a lack of intellectual capacity. He also didn't romanticize them. With the exception of the self-committed, who he saw as unfortunate victims of circumstance rather than criminals, he described the drunkards and tramps in the Workhouse as worthless. But in the very same annual report where he expressed that sentiment he wrote, "There is no more hopeful class, as a whole, than the prisoners of the Work House."

Perhaps it was the challenge. Jesus became "poor for our sakes," he would later write, and "we must see Him and minister to Him in the persons both of the evil and the good."

But French had to act fast when it came to Workhouse inmates. They were never there for very long, generally only ten days to a few months, and it didn't give him much time to get to know them or find a way to help. But what was such a success with the patients at the Lunatic Asylum turned out to be an even bigger hit with the inmates at the Workhouse.

When French began his mission in 1872, the Workhouse was without a library of any kind. It wasn't that the inmates were uninterested in reading. "I have given over one thousand papers to the inmates, and could have distributed three times as many," French insisted, "for they seem anxious for reading-matter." But installing a library proved a harder task than it was at the Lunatic Asylum. He started with only a bookcase in the chapel he shared with the Catholic priests. It would be another six years before he was finally able to open a small library. French never explained what the holdup was, perhaps out of discretion. These were the degraded souls who should be spending all their time learning to love work and near-starving, the commissioners felt. The idea of any of them curling up and losing themselves in a good book may have struck the commissioners as an outrage. But in the Workhouse library's first two years they went from getting twelve readers a week to 1,400. In 1882 French would triumphantly announce that "in the Work-House, whose inmates stand lowest in the scale of intellect and of moral character," the books had been checked out 50,000 times in the previous four years.

It couldn't have helped that while French was in the midst of trying to give the Workhouse inmates a library, the Great Depression was in full swing. The total admissions in the Workhouse jumped from 21,882 in 1871 to 33,757 in 1875, a figure that included a large number of self-committed. (As a reminder, the able-bodied poor were no longer welcome at the Almshouse, and if they had no place else to go they had to commit themselves to the Workhouse). During that period a smaller amount of money from the city had to be stretched to cope with swelling numbers of inmates. French continued to do everything he could to be of service to the men and women of the Workhouse. After they were discharged, he tried to help them find employment and wrote letters of recommendation whenever he had the opportunity.

French was once again called before the Committee of Direction of the New York Protestant Episcopal City Mission Society. This time it was not about talking to a newspaper reporter, it was about his spending. French had apparently been having financial difficulties of his own. The committee sent him a note: "Having learned with great surprise . . . from various outside sources that you are in the constant habit of borrowing money from both clergy & laity & that you are largely in debt thereby very seriously imposing yourself & especially the church & this Society." The committee was concerned that his borrowing would cast discredit on the Society. French was asked to make a list of his debts and to appear before them to explain. "Your continuance as an employee of this Society will depend on your prompt & full response."

French often carried bags of candies and oranges with him to give out as he walked up and down the Island and in and out of the institutions, visiting with inmates. To a man who has been breaking rocks all day, whose only crime might have been homelessness, or a woman suffering from anxiety and depression and who has been sitting in a cell for months or years, both of whom had been living in a near-constant state of deprivation, a simple orange or bag of sweets from someone whose eyes expressed concern and not disgust may have been one of the few gestures they experienced as genuinely charitable.

French paid for these small gifts out of his own pocket, and his debts included a hefty grocery bill. He also absorbed the cost of the paper and stamps for his letters of recommendation, and he occasionally helped discharged inmates with car-fare and night lodgings. In addition to the grocery bill, French had taken out a loan from a fellow priest, and he also had a long-overdue coal bill. The largest debt, however, was not his, but his previous employer's, and everything was eventually smoothed out.

French could have gotten help with his family's coal supply from the Department of Public Charities and Correction, who distributed coal to the poor for the asking (with demonstration of need). Close to 4,000 tons of coal were given out that year to over 10,000 families. But it was inconceivable that French would ever apply. It would not do for him to appear as if he was one step away from the Almshouse himself.

While French was struggling to pay his coal bill Josephine Shaw Lowell was doing everything she could to abolish the practice of supplying coal to the poor, as well as every other form of what was called "outdoor relief." Outdoor relief simply meant any aid given to the poor outside of an institution. Lowell was a strict proponent of the idea that institutionalization was the best way to help the poor. According to Joan Waugh in *Unsentimental Reformer: The Life of Josephine Shaw Lowell*, the effort to eliminate outdoor relief "struck down two evils for the price of one: it eliminated a source of political patronage for the machine and a corrupting influence for the poor."

The source of political patronage was the Department of Public Charities and Correction, whose staff was appointed based on connections, not expertise, and who in turn hired their friends to work in all the prisons, asylums, hospitals, and other institutions they oversaw. The corrupting influence refers to the rationale for having a Workhouse in the first place, and it was the same logic Lowell used when commenting on the unfortunate Julia Deems, whose infant daughter died when they were shoved out into the cold by Julia's drunken husband. If we give the poor handouts, all we teach them is to expect more handouts. While New Yorkers were in the middle of the Great Depression and 25 percent of the city's workers had found themselves unemployed over the winter of 1873–74, Lowell would ultimately succeed in eliminating outdoor relief by 1876, except for coal disbursements and cash stipends to the blind.

Lowell did not intend to abandon the poor, however. In 1879, while French was writing how "good and evil alternate in quick succession," on Blackwell's Island, Lowell was strenuously pushing for a Workhouse alternative for women only, an institution that would be less punitive and more reformatory. It was much needed, but Lowell went rather far. She proposed establishing reformatories, "to which all women under thirty, when arrested for misdemeanors, or upon the birth of a second illegitimate child, should be committed for very long periods (not as a punishment, but for the same reason that the insane are sent to an asylum), and where they should be subject to such a physical, moral and intellectual training as would re-create them."

She thought the problem was that they needed "to be taught to be women; they must be induced to love that which is good and pure, and to wish to resemble it; they must learn all household duties; they must learn to enjoy work; they must have a future to look forward to; and they must be cured, both body and soul, before they can be safely trusted to face the world again."

Lowell had come up with this radical solution after reading the *Tenth Annual Report of the State Board of Charities*, which dealt with the causes of pauperism. She decided that "one of the most important and most dangerous causes of the increase of crime, pauperism, and insanity is the unrestrained liberty allowed to vagrant and degraded women." Later in 1879, on November 24, a former Workhouse inmate who signed her name as Miss Morgan wrote a letter to the editor of the *New York Herald*. In her letter she referred to the "State Lady," who was almost certainly Josephine Shaw Lowell. Morgan wanted Lowell to understand that life on the inside was very different than what visitors like Lowell saw on Workhouse tours.

How could Lowell truly know who they were and the conditions they were living under, Miss Morgan asked, when visitors were forbidden from speaking to the prisoners? The inmates were not all immoral and unprincipled criminals, as portrayed, but "hard working, ignorant beings, who, thrown out of employment, are committed for a month of correction, and are forced to associate . . . with some poor creatures who are so depraved they know not right from wrong." To make matters worse, the people hired to look after them made no effort to distinguish them. "The matrons, from having so mixed a class of prisoners to deal with are hard and exacting, showing no sympathy, and they assume a tyrannical bearing to all alike, saying that no innocent women would be sent there."

In reality it was as easy to get an innocent person sent to the Workhouse as it was to get a sane person committed to an asylum. In 1880 two people found a doctor who was willing to say that their elderly Aunt Delia was a drunkard. On the basis of this and their corroborating testimony a judge sentenced Delia to six months in the Workhouse. While she was imprisoned the nephew and his wife sold everything Delia had for $1,200. The superintendent of the Workhouse, who could find no evidence of a lifetime of drinking, wrote to the judge to ask why he had committed her. A trial was held, with French as a character witness for Delia, and Delia's nephew was found guilty of perjury and sentenced to four years of hard labor at the state prison.

The "State Lady . . . makes her visits occasionally," Miss Morgan wrote, "and thinks the food is good enough for them, when it is served as though they were animals, and often so bad as to cause riots and desperation. The women are worked hard and half fed." Morgan was not exaggerating. The daily cost per Workhouse inmate was generally 15 cents, almost half of what it was for the patients at the Lunatic Asylum who, everyone conceded, were starving.

Miss Morgan begged the *Herald*'s readers to see that the Workhouse, "that so-called institution 'for charities and correction,'" was in reality the very exemplification of misclassification. "I suggest that if a woman is bad enough to steal the Penitentiary is the place for her; that if she is committed for drinking—and arrested while in the worst stage—she should be placed in the hospital until she is herself again."

But while Morgan and Lowell agreed on what the Workhouse was not, they did not agree on what the Workhouse could be. While Lowell would concede that inmates were "treated with a certain brutality of manner by some of the paid employees of the department," nonetheless, "this institution should be used as a reformatory for the men and women committed to it, or should at least be a place of punishment. At present it is not even the last; there is not any strict enforcement of discipline, nor is the amount of work required sufficient to have a deterrent effect on the inmates after a first commitment." Lowell was another in a long line of investigators to recognize that the Workhouse did not turn out as reformers had dreamed.

Not long after Miss Morgan's letter, Rev. French was given help with the mission on Blackwell's Island. In the ten years he'd been serving on the Island, the number of people being committed there had increased 20 percent yearly, and French was sixty-seven years old. In 1881 Reverend Jerome B. Morse joined him on his daily trip across the river. The institutions were divided up, and responsibility for the Workhouse was transferred to the younger priest. Morse quickly became frustrated by the same question that had always weighed on French: did anything he did to help make a difference? French understood all too well. "Twelve years of labor in these institutions," he would write two years later, "have been a trial to faith which none can imagine," except those who have been there and put in the time.

In a couple of years Morse assumed a more accepting attitude. "The moral results are for the most part invisible, and, like the water-marks beneath the written page that are only seen when held up to the light, will not be known till seen in the light of eternity." By 1886 he was positively giddy. "I am glad to report that this last year has been my best year," he wrote. He'd had a lot of success mediating between prisoners and their family, friends, and former employers. The women he'd been sending to the Faith Home upon discharge were finding work.

Morse was especially happy with the new superintendent of the Workhouse, the Reverend William R. Stocking, whose first day was January 1, 1886. Stocking had immediately established a new temperance organization and already thousands had signed on. It wasn't that the priests had a moralistic, anti-alcohol stance. It was the destructive aftermath, which the priests witnessed up close daily. Many of the people in the Workhouse wouldn't be there if they hadn't done something stupid or worse while they were drinking, things that they would never do sober. The priests were simply trying to make sure the inmates never did anything to compel their return. Not a lot was known then (or arguably now) about how to help people to stop drinking, and Morse was glad that the new superintendent was at least willing to try to do something to accomplish one of the goals the institution had been built for: reform.

Morse's 1886 report was bursting with optimism. "I find that time and experience in my special field are my best capital to work with. Really, a month seems to be now as good as my first year." A few good months were all he would get. Not long after writing those cheery words Morse died unexpectedly, on November 2. He was fifty-eight years old.

But Rev. Stocking, too, was full of the feeling that he might be able to turn things around for the largest population of what was seen as yet another mismanaged institution. The son of missionaries, Stocking had been born in Persia (present-day Iran), and he was only forty-two years old when he assumed his role as the superintendent of the Blackwell's Island Workhouse. The commissioners, anxious for new management and a new take on the problem, had put their faith in the relatively young priest. It was a bit of a gamble.

Stocking had no background in penal management. He'd resigned his position as pastor at White Oaks Church in Massachusetts in order to take the job, and his sole training was the few days he spent at the New York State Reformatory in Elmira. Stocking believed the Elmira Reformatory was getting at least some things right—Josephine Shaw Lowell also thought this—and his time there gave him a lot of ideas. But he saw almost at once that he wouldn't be able to implement them at the Workhouse.

Stocking, too, had come to believe that classification was crucial to reform. But in his first year, 11,978 men and 9,649 women were admitted to the Workhouse. He soon grasped what every other superintendent had:

that the Workhouse was routinely overrun with hordes of people who were in and out far too quickly for effective classification. Worse, "the class of keepers and employees was of a low order because politics had much to do with their appointment." Miss Morgan had not exaggerated. Stocking was shocked by their brutality.

But in this one respect, Stocking would succeed where the Lunatic Asylum resident physician Dr. William Strew had failed. In his first six months, Stocking had successfully "gotten rid of several incompetent officials" including the deputy superintendent, four keepers, the night watchman, and the head matron. Unlike Strew, Stocking was able to proclaim that "the Commissioners stood by me faithfully," which may have been a testament to his persuasive skills, but more likely it was an indication of just how anxious the commissioners were to make an active show at reform.

Months before Stocking was hired, the Irish American, Catholic mayor William Grace, who would accept the gift of the Statue of Liberty from France that same year, had replaced Commissioner and President of the Department of Public Charities and Correction Jacob Hess with Dr. Charles E. Simmons, someone whom Grace saw as more a man of science than a politician. Reformer Josephine Shaw Lowell's name had been bandied about as well, but Mayor Grace thought "a woman could not know anything about the prisons" and went with Simmons. Hess had lobbied hard to keep his position, but Grace wanted change (just not too much change; he wasn't progressive enough to appoint a woman).

Dr. Simmons hired Stocking. This explains how someone with such a sweet temperament ever came to take charge of the Workhouse in the first place. In his inaugural report to Simmons and the other commissioners, Stocking wrote, "In my dealings with these people, it has been my aim to be, in the first place, Just. In the second place, Firm. In the third place, Kind." No Workhouse superintendent before Stocking had ever written such gentle lines. Junius Henri Browne would say the superintendents on Blackwell's were generally "hard, unfeeling and tyrannical, and not unfrequently brutal and cruel to the last degree. Their position is not calculated to develop the sensibilities or refine the sentiments, and they do not enter upon their duties with any surplus of charity or tenderness. . . . If they were fine or gentle natures, they would not be there; for saints do not gravitate to the custodianship of prisons and poor-houses." Stocking was especially hopeful about his new matron, Mrs. Sarah Holt, whom he saw as his partner-in-reform.

In his first year, Stocking had new bathtubs installed on the women's side, and then he gave them an area in the backyard in which to congregate after their bath. On the men's side he rearranged the use of some of the rooms so that they could reduce the number of men in the larger cells from thirty-six and twenty-four to twelve. He also promoted a worker who'd spent time trying to educate inmates to the position of Workhouse Teacher, and established a Workhouse school.

One morning an inmate named Miller came to Stocking in his office. "I wish you would do me a great favor Superintendent."

"What is it?"

"Will you put my name on the list of those to be discharged this noon, instead of tonight?"

When Stocking asked why, Miller explained that he'd been arrested for the first time, for drunkenness, and he was owed wages by his employer in the city. If he got there too late to collect he'd end up wandering the streets until morning as he had no place to stay and no money.

What about your family? Stocking asked.

They were in Georgia.

Stocking looked at the man's file. "Were you in the unpleasantness we had between the north and the south a few years ago?" he asked, referring politely to the Civil War.

"Yes," Miller answered.

"Were you at the Battle of Winchester, September 19th?"

"I sure was!"

Stocking, a Union soldier with the Thirty-Fourth Regiment of the

Massachusetts Infantry, had been shot in the foot at that battle. He was limping off the battlefield when he came across a fellow Union soldier escorting a captured Confederate soldier from the Second Georgia Infantry to the rear. The three men talked briefly and the Confederate prisoner turned out to be a very likable and good-natured young man. Stocking impulsively asked the prisoner if he wouldn't mind helping him walk. "Don't mind if I do Yank!" the man answered. Stocking handed his gun and knapsack to his comrade, leaned on the Georgian's shoulder, and together they made their way back to the Union camp. The prisoner's name was Miller. Stocking looked up at the inmate before him. Could this be the same man? "Were you captured in the fight that day?" He wasn't. "But I had a brother who was made a prisoner on that day." Stocking later wrote the brother, who'd survived the war and remembered the day he helped a supposed enemy off the battlefield.

Stocking returned the favor by making sure his brother was put on an early boat off the Island. After that, Stocking made this standard practice for all inmates (previously only prisoners with long-term sentences were sent home early). On the last day of an inmate's sentence, "instead of making them work all day, and sending them out on the last boat in the afternoon, without supper, (many having no where to go)," they would now give inmates "their supper and breakfast, and send them forth by the first boat in the morning, when the sun is high and hope is nigh, and the chance to find a place and employment is much greater."

Stocking finished that first year with two primary obsessions: rounders and temperance. At the end of 1887, he surveyed the inmates who remained in the Workhouse and asked if they'd been sentenced there before. Eighteen percent of the men and 58 percent of the women confessed that they had.

The fact that there were more female rounders than male (or perhaps the women were merely more truthful) was interpreted in several ways. Many saw it as proof that women were less capable of improving their lives. One Workhouse superintendent said the rounder statistics were "an

interesting corroboration of the saying that after a woman falls there is little hope for her reformation." Others saw it as evidence of the crippling bias
towards women from both the criminal justice system and general society,
which hampered their reformation. "A woman, if once committed to the
Island, is rarely forgotten," the Women's Prison Association reported, "either by the officials or by her fellow prisoners. She has not an equal chance
with men. If she has been sent up as a prostitute, there is no way open for
her but the street."

It wasn't that women were less capable of reform, many argued. Society wouldn't let them reform themselves, and the Workhouse was no help.
"Her incarceration has done her no good," the New York Charity Organization wrote, "for if it be her first imprisonment she is detained but five
days. She has no opportunity to learn a useful occupation, and she returns,
perforce, to her previous method of living. If she is fined, she must in some
manner earn the money thus lost by the fine, and she earns it in the same
way as before and, possibly, also by thievery."

In her 1879 report "One Means of Preventing Pauperism," Lowell
quoted Dr. Elisha Harris, the Corresponding Secretary of the New York
Prison Association. "In one county I saw three girls, who had been tramping all summer as leaders of a band of tramping boys. . . . When they wept,
as though penitent, and asked who cared for them, the sheriff and his assistants seemed to regard them as objects of derision and sport. . . . In another jail, I found that a sheriff . . . had wantonly assaulted and degraded
numerous young women prisoners; and, when sheriff in 1871 and 1872, had
utterly brutalized three young girls."

Nellie Bly herself spent time with women who had recently been arrested, and published an article in 1888 titled "Why Don't Women Reform?" Part of the problem, many of the women she spoke to conceded,
was alcohol. But throwing them into a place with habitual criminals was
no solution. "We are not so bad at first, but every time we go back we get
worse," one woman told her. "Then, you see, the police get to know us,
and it's no use trying. They run us in just for the sake of having a case.

Then they lie about us." Bly would point out that when a woman disputed an arresting officer's version of events, the same arresting officer was the one assigned to investigate her claim. Even if she tried to reform, another woman said, "the very police who have pulled me in would jeer me on the streets." Then, echoing her fellow detainee, "once the police know you, you are done for." Bly, mistakenly thinking that the toil of a regular job was part of the problem, said to one woman that work "isn't so hard after a while." The woman gravely answered, "There are things hundreds of times harder than work."

At the end of her article Bly wrote of two findings that had made the greatest impression on her: "First, the utter uselessness of the modern form of punishment. Second, that the majority of misery results from cheap drinks."

Josephine Shaw Lowell's suggestion of a reformatory for women alone, and for longer and broader sentencing, came in part from recognizing this bias towards women and she offered this as a practical solution. Both Josephine Shaw Lowell and the Women's Prison Association saw the women's reformatory they both championed not as punitive (or not entirely punitive, anyway), but as a place to give women the same chance men had to change their ways and get a fresh start at a new life.

It's not clear how Stocking viewed the gender difference in the rounder totals, only that he was committed to reducing their numbers altogether, and he had an idea he believed would help: cumulative sentencing. Instead of having people go in and out of the Workhouse for ten days at a time, over and over and over, "these people, even for intoxication, should have perhaps ten days at first, one month for second offense, three months for the third, and so on up to a year."

He argued that short sentences that were constantly repeated by a large group of people reduced the Workhouse to a house of detention only, making reformation, the ideal he hoped to finally realize, impossible. But he also appealed to less noble concerns. There was the expense of arrest, trial, conviction, transportation, and then processing, feeding, clothing, and housing those continually sentenced there. Due to the short sentences, the inmates were rarely there long enough to provide useful and productive labor on the Island or even cover the costs of their care. Cumulative sentencing would neatly address all these ills.

Hand in hand with cumulative sentencing was his goal of "having the law changed so that a Police Magistrate *can not* discharge, at pleasure, persons whom he has committed to the Work House." Under the current system, inmates were free to go around the Workhouse superintendent and petition the police justices directly for discharge. The police justices, who kept poor records and would often "recklessly" sentence the same people sometimes ten or twenty times or more in the same year, were so casual about discharging inmates that occasionally the same people showed up in court before their previous sentence had expired. "If any are to be discharged before their time," Stocking argued, "it should be only those whose record of behavior and work has been nearly perfect, and who can go directly from here to work awaiting them outside." And that, he believed, was a decision that should be made by commissioners of the Department, who would be advised by a committee who had examined the merits of the individual case.

Stocking's second passion was temperance. Bly's conclusion about cheap drink at the end of her article mirrored Stocking's views. "Our books show that fully 30 percent of those who have taken the pledge in our Temperance Society, have not as yet returned to the Work House." A 30 percent reduction in recidivism is an impressive accomplishment, if true. By the end of Stocking's first year, 1,612 men and 1,060 women stood up and recited "I promise to abstain from the use of all intoxicating drinks as a beverage, and to discountenance their use by others. So help me God."

Life on the Island that year was both a happy and sad one for Stocking. On November 9, 1887, his son Charles Parsons was born. But the joy of new life was quickly shattered by the death of his oldest son, eleven-year-old Lyman, one month later. Stocking's tone in his next annual report grew dark. "The class of people who come to the Work-House are perhaps more difficult to deal with than any others who are under restraint. . . . Their misdemeanors and petty crimes are so insidious and so thoroughly mean and contemptible." His new matron, Mrs. Sarah Holt, who he had hoped would spearhead change on the women's side, had quit after only six months. In a letter addressed to the mayor, she proclaimed that reformation in the present Workhouse was "well nigh impossible," and that "as a Christian people, we are guilty before God of the appalling sin of neglect of our most precious charge, the poor and defenseless, in so much as they have not been protected from open-faced prostitution, though entitled to the same rights of protection as the refined demand and enjoy."

Stocking was now beginning to think that the only way to fix their problems was to start with a clean slate. Just shut the Workhouse down and try again. The Workhouse as it was then "constituted and arranged, cannot be made in any true sense a reformatory." Under the current system he was forced to treat the destitute, who were "not in any legal sense criminals," nearly the same "as those committed by the courts."

The way Stocking now envisioned it, a "truly reformative" institution would be "located on a large farm—where, in addition to plenty of out-door work, there should be taught a variety of trades and useful occupations— and from which all discharged prisoners should be sent to some definite and regular work provided for them. . . . There is no doubt that these people should be made to work, and to *work hard*—but at the same time their work should be so arranged as to prepare them to earn a honest living."

A few months before the death of Stocking's son, Josephine Shaw Lowell submitted the findings of her most recent investigation into Workhouse abuses. She'd put off making a report the previous year because Stocking and his new matron, Mrs. Holt, had only just started in their new positions. Lowell wanted to give them both a chance to effect change. But now the matron was gone, convinced that reform at the present Workhouse was out of the question. Stocking, too, "is also filled with dismay and horror," she wrote, "at the evils inseparable from the massing of offenders of almost every age and every degree of vicious degradation, in a building where classification is a physical impossibility, and under officers so few in number that even a pretense of discipline is a farce."

Lowell's attitude towards the poor was actually beginning to soften. "If the working people had all they ought to have," she wrote to her sister-in-law in 1889, "we should not have the paupers and criminals. It is better to save them before they go under, than to spend your life fishing them out."

It seemed from her 1887 report, where she described people filing into the Workhouse "in two long, hopeless trains of degraded men and women," that her compassion had truly expanded. "The contrast between the decrepit and broken-down old men, tottering to their graves, worn out with dissipation and suffering, and the boys of seventeen and eighteen, weak and coarse, just entering on the same destructive career, and utterly indifferent to their own degradation and careless of their future, is heart-breaking."

Lowell wrote about how an assistant matron at the Workhouse, "told me of four young girls, who are now constantly returning to the workhouse under sentence for disorderly conduct, all of whom had (on their first conviction) there made the acquaintance of a woman undergoing sentence for keeping a Chinese dive." The woman, who had since been discharged, met the girls "at the Twenty-Sixth Street dock, and took them to her 'dive,' where she drugged them. They were only about seventeen years of age at that time," but they had fallen and now their fates were inexorably sealed.

Lowell ended her report with the appalling fact that in the previous year 351 boys and 79 girls under twenty years old had been incarcerated in the Workhouse. The fact that there was no place in New York City "for a boy or girl over sixteen, guilty of a misdemeanor or arrested as a vagrant . . . except the work-house or penitentiary," made what she saw as "the crying need of adult reformatories in New York City" absolutely indisputable.

Stocking continued to point to alcohol as one of the largest contributing factors. "The records of the criminal courts in this State and in this country show that fully eighty per cent of those arrested and convicted as violators of the law owe their misfortune and sin to the inflamed condition of their passions brought about through intoxicating drinks." That same figure continues to be quoted today, well over a hundred years later. According to the National Council on Alcoholism and Drug Dependence, "Alcohol and drugs are implicated in an estimated 80% of offenses leading to incarceration in the United States such as domestic violence, driving while intoxicated, property offenses, drug offenses, and public-order offenses."

That spring the editors of the *New York World* decided to see if they could make lightning strike twice. Seven months after assigning Nellie Bly to get herself committed to the Lunatic Asylum in order to report undercover, they assigned a young reporter named William P. Rogers to get himself convicted of a minor crime so that he could write a similar exposé about the Workhouse.

A WORKHOUSE EXPOSÉ AND LAWRENCE DUNPHY

Superintendent of the Blackwell's Island Workhouse from 1889 to 1896

———————◆———————

On April 27, 1888, Rogers had one drink, feigned intoxication, and managed to make enough of a nuisance of himself to get arrested for disorderly conduct. He couldn't make bail, he told the police justice at the Jefferson Market Courthouse, so the very next day he was loaded onto the steamer *Thomas S. Brennan* (named for one of the commissioners) and shipped to Blackwell's Island. His article titled "A Month in the Workhouse" came out on June 10.

"For a man who has never experienced what it is to be cribbed, cabined and confined," Rogers wrote, "it is no light matter to be subjected to the machine-like direction of those who appear to be selected for the discharge of their duties principally because of their stolid indifference to all the claims and instincts of humanity."

His experience echoed Bly's in many ways. The newly admitted were bathed one after another in the same bathwater in eight shared bathtubs. Rogers was lucky enough to be one of the first, but he could see how "the water would, in a short time, become somewhat thick, if not lively." And Rogers claimed to have never seen a piece of soap during his entire incarceration.

He was put in Cell No. 39 on the top tier, where he was locked up for the night with thirty-two men and only wooden buckets to serve as a bathroom. Rogers dryly noted, "so that it will not be difficult for the intelligent reader to imagine how poisonous the atmosphere must become before morning." A bucket of water was also placed in the cell for drinking purposes, but this, too, became "positively loathsome" by the morning.

Although Rogers tried to infuse his report with the horror of it all, at times he sounds like a privileged kid who was getting a thrill out of slumming it. "Every evening after supper," he wrote, there was a hunt for vermin in the cells, and on "Sundays there is a grand slaughter."

He called the self-committed, who went to the Workhouse when money, whiskey, and food ran out, "otherwise useless loafers," which was the prevailing opinion of his time. A man died in one of the dark cells during Rogers' incarceration, and the night watchmen told him it was not an isolated case. It happened because there was only one night watchman assisted by two male prisoners for the entire Workhouse, and anyone in a dark cell was routinely left alone until the morning.

As bad as the food at the Lunatic Asylum was, the food at the Workhouse was worse. Rogers made it sound utterly putrid and unpalatable. Meat destined for the Almshouse and Workhouse smelled so bad that "when it was brought off the boat every man held his nose." The Almshouse managers had the good sense to send their share of the meat back, but the Workhouse managers kept their allotment.

Rogers saved his strongest criticism for the bakery. Men with open sores who slept on floors stained with tobacco juice and other filth, and who were "so thoroughly infested with vermin" that no one would go near them, were the ones "who make the bread for all the hospitals and other institutions under the charge of the Commissioners of Charities and Correction."

Roger was moved to write, "I have felt strongly since, that whatever rights the city may have to impose punishment for the infraction of one of its ordinances, it certainly can have no right thus to sow in men's systems the germs of disease."

Commissioner Brennan called on Stocking to respond. Stocking must have felt at least somewhat resentful. He customarily took part in assessing every inmate, and he'd tried to show Rogers a little kindness. Rogers had come to the Workhouse with a black eye, and "in such a dilapidated condition, that I at once marked him for light work at the Storehouse, which would give him an opportunity to get over the effect of his debauch." From there, all Stocking could do was deny Rogers' claims. Men sent to the bakery were bathed first, "and we are always particularly careful not to send men with sores or ulcers." And "as to our facilities for cleanliness, they might be made more adequate," Stocking conceded, but he also expressed the hope that everything would be better once their new building was ready. There was one denial he could not make, however. "As to deaths in the padded cell, they certainly do occur occasionally." But men were put there "by order of the Physician, and while there, are under his special care, and are visited by the night man on duty in the hospital, at regular intervals." Stocking clearly believed what he was writing, but it was almost certainly untrue.

There was no outcry after Rogers' article, and no grand-jury investigation. Although part of the reason was that Rogers was not as skilled as Bly in crafting a story, the larger explanation is, unlike the women in the Lunatic Asylum, Workhouse inmates were not seen as innocent victims, and were therefore undeserving of sympathy. They had it coming. Even if Rogers had been a great writer, what he witnessed was never going to be able to compete with defenseless women in a Lunatic Asylum being abused by evil nurses who were supposed to be caring and kind. The prison keepers were just doing their job, and life inside the Workhouse was supposed to be harrowing.

ON JANUARY 21, 1889, Stocking's wife gave birth on the Island to a baby daughter, Isabella Caroline, who "came to us at the end of a stormy night," Stocking wrote. He also thought to note, "That Monday brought one hundred and forty-five admissions to the Workhouse."

A few months later, Stocking was ordered to switch places with Lawrence

Dunphy, the superintendent of the smaller Branch Workhouse on Hart Island (another island further north), who'd been in that position since 1876. It was a move that can only be seen as a demotion. The number of inmates passing through the Branch Workhouse yearly was generally less than 1,500. More than twenty times that number were admitted to the Workhouse on Blackwell's. On Stocking's last night on Blackwell's Island, which also happened to be his forty-fifth birthday, a farewell temperance meeting was held, with forty-eight new members taking the pledge. It was the most meaningful way Rev. Stocking could have said goodbye. The following evening, his first on Hart Island, was marked a little differently. On April 1, a prisoner in Barracks No. 3 was murdered, and Stocking began his tenure with an inquest.

Although the Women's Prison Association had always been admiring of Stocking's efforts at the Workhouse, in their next report they were positively ecstatic about Dunphy. "The discipline at this place is excellent," they raved. Both the prisoners and the attendants were in "mortal terror of Superintendent Dunphy," who ruled the Workhouse with a militaristic fist. It was exactly what the place needed, they felt. "The women march to their meals, which they eat without a word."

Dunphy was even more strict about discharging the self-committed, who could no longer simply check themselves out at will but had to show evidence of work waiting for them on the outside. When Mayor Abram Hewitt wrote the commissioners on behalf of one particular inmate who was unsuccessful in obtaining a release, Dunphy continued to withhold his recommendation for a discharge. The commissioner's office wrote again, this time asking Dunphy to explain his reason. "He spends his time, when out, in draining beer kegs set outside of saloons, and is an annoyance to the city." Everyone, except the people who had to go back to the mayor, was thrilled. Even Rev. French was enthusiastic about Dunphy. "Though just and kind[,] he is a strict disciplinarian. It may be truly said of him that he 'is the right man in the right place.'"

For the rest of his life Stocking worried that his transfer may have been partly political, and that may have been true. Although Dunphy didn't bow to political pressure, Stocking was an activist. He repeatedly wrote Mayor Hewitt to complain about a common practice at the police stations, whose basements were used, legally, as lodging houses for vagrants. Sometimes, "the Police Officer in charge of the Station" when feeling "out of sorts . . . will send a batch of men and women to the Court, simply because he is tired of having so many lodgers." There they'd be charged en masse with disorderly conduct and sentenced to the Workhouse for three months. The police were creating a growing group of now unfairly labeled "ex-cons" and Stocking wanted them released and their unjust sentences vacated.

When police justices discharged a large number of male prisoners, who also happened to be voters, just before the city and state elections, Stocking complained so loudly he was called to Albany to testify. He also lectured to community groups like the YMCA, whenever the opportunity arose, about the need for cumulative sentencing, which was seen as yet another criticism of the police justices.

The truth was Stocking really was a bit of a soft touch, especially compared to the no-nonsense Dunphy. When young men were sentenced to the Workhouse, Stocking tried to impose at least some measure of classification by assigning them to clerical work in the office. This kept them away from the "rougher crowd." He also came up with other ways to send discharged inmates back out into the world "with a hope for better things." First-time inmates, for instance, left the Island with "their clothing mended and shoes repaired . . . so that they might go out with self respect." Those who had been "faithful in their work for several months," were sometimes presented with a real prize: a brand new pair of shoes.

Stocking's sympathetic nature almost cost him his job even sooner. A woman who'd never been committed before and who'd just had a baby was sentenced to the Workhouse. "In a few days she became distracted, almost crazy, to see her child," Stocking wrote. Mrs. Holt tried to comfort her, but "as time went on the condition of the woman grew worse, and Mrs. Holt fearing that she would become insane asked me if I could not arrange in some way so that she could see her child." There was a rowboat crossing at Seventy-Sixth Street every hour. Stocking told Mrs. Holt to have the woman dressed in her own clothing "as if she were to be discharged," and he would row her over to see her baby himself. From there they'd take the Second Avenue El downtown together to see her child on Hester Street, on the Lower East Side.

A thunderstorm struck just when they got within a few blocks of her sister-in-law's apartment, where her baby was staying. Stocking didn't immediately suspect a problem when the woman went into another room to change out of her wet clothes. After a few minutes he asked after her. She's not ready, he was told. "After a longer wait I insisted on going to the back room." He'd waited too long. The woman had climbed out of a window and could now be anywhere in the city.

A relative of Stocking's put him in touch with a detective agency and he was assured that they'd put their best men on the case. "Alone, somewhat crestfallen, I returned to my duties at the Workhouse." The detectives managed to intercept a note from the woman to her husband. The two were to meet up downtown, in a wholesale warehouse area. The detectives sent the letter back on its way to the husband and contacted Stocking. Taking a keeper he could trust, Stocking rowed back to Manhattan to join the detectives. They divided the area to be searched, with the detectives going one way and Stocking and his keeper another. "We tramped for several hours in the dark, damp, fog filled alleys and byways of lower New York," and they were about to give up when Stocking spotted a woman wrapped in a black cape. He went over to her himself, and took hold of the arm of his escaped prisoner.

It must have been a quiet and cheerless ride back uptown. When they got to the landing at Seventy-Sixth Street Stocking had to blow a horn to call another boat. As they rowed back over the turbulent river to Blackwell's, the woman sobbed. Don't put me in a dark cell, she pleaded. But Stocking had as much to lose as she did if any word of the episode got out. Never say a word of this to anyone, he told her, and I won't punish you. "I gave each of the detectives ten dollars," he wrote later, "and charged it to Experience."

Stocking would continue his compassionate approach at his new post on Hart Island, although he wouldn't remain there long either. One of his first acts was to create a reformatory for the younger inmates, which would finally keep them away from the more hardened criminals. In 1890, two years after Stocking began his work there, while the Women's Prison Association was praising Dunphy, and deservedly so, Stocking's youngest daughter Isabella Caroline died on Hart Island on March 12. Once more Stocking would climb into a rowboat, this time to make a trip to leave "the little body near that of her brother Lyman." His wife would follow their daughter only a few months later when she died on August 17. When he was offered the position as the superintendent for the Fairview Home for Friendless Children in upstate New York the following year, he accepted.

Stocking's call for cumulative sentences meanwhile had been taken up by the Women's Prison Association and others. The Women's Prison Association also called for change within the Department of Public Charities and Correction. They'd made what was quite a daring suggestion for the time, "that women commissioners would greatly benefit these unfortunate members of society." It was one thing to put a woman in charge of a charitable institution. Managing prisons was strictly men's work. But they had an even bigger revamp in mind. "Now the same three men care for all, for the drunkard and disorderly person, for the pauper, the insane, the blind, the idiot, for little babies, and hardened criminals," who were all conveyed "in the same boat to the same islands. Thus the innocent and the guilty associate, more or less, until their return." The Women's Prison Association was joining the call for a major change which reformers had been trying to advance for some time: the separation of the administration of public charity from that of incarceration and correction.

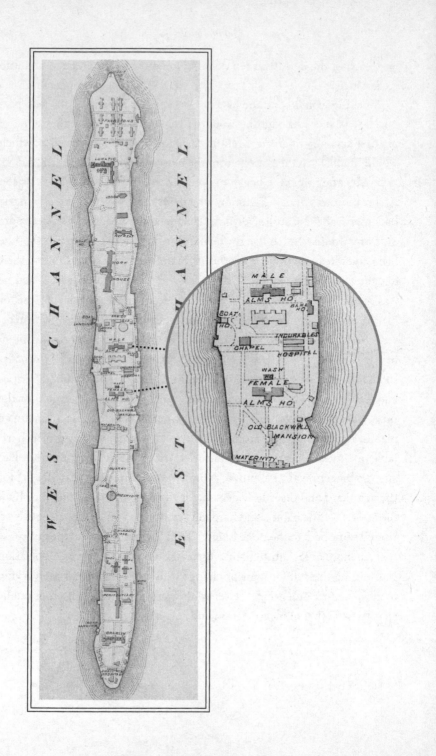

⌦ III ⌫

THE ALMSHOUSE

———◆———

COMPLETED IN 1848, TO HOUSE THE POOR
AND DISABLED OF NEW YORK CITY

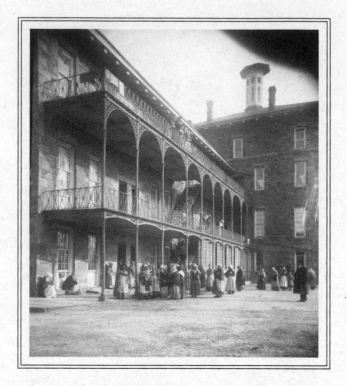

THE ALMSHOUSE COMPLEX
The End of the Line for Many

———————◆———————

REV. FRENCH ALWAYS looked back on his time in North Carolina as something of a failure. "I came out of the mountains of North Carolina greatly broken up," he admitted. He'd spent three years helping to establish a new mission in a remote region called Valle Crucis, and his efforts had gotten off to a disheartening start. As he approached Greensboro, French came across a mob on their way to the hanging of a black man. "After living awhile in a slave state, I ceased from feeling any surprise at [the] want of sympathy," he recorded in his journal; nonetheless later that night at dinner, when talk of the hanging came up, he "was much shocked at some unfeeling remarks made at table about negroes, by two young lawyers, and a lady of the house."

There were also never enough funds for the monastic community he was expected to establish. When a young postulant arrived and wrote the bishop criticizing French for how he spent and borrowed money, essentially accusing him of running the mission into the ground, French came to believe that his bishop had lost faith in him. He resigned to give a new man a shot at doing better. That man would last a year.

On Blackwell's Island French had a second chance, and with a mission that was far more dangerous than anything he had encountered in North Carolina. The ferry rides themselves could be harrowing. Before being transported to New York's potter's field on Hart Island, dead bodies from Blackwell's (and elsewhere) were placed on vessels in unsealed, often-broken coffins, described as "not liquid tight." The corpses would sometimes wait on the dock for hours, rotting in the sun, dripping next to foodstuffs like the carcasses of sheep, which had only a torn cheese cloth to protect them from whatever was leaking out of those coffins before being delivered to Blackwell's Island, where they'd be consumed by inmates and staff alike.

A *New York Times* reporter wrote how the people on Blackwell's, and "particularly the old men and women" of the Almshouse, would see those steamboats and "shrink back into darker shaded corners and press away from the river banks and look with terror and awe at the big black heap upon the forward deck. Some of their friends are there. . . . The next time the boat goes up they may make a part of this black cargo. They know it and shrink away."

And yet for French every time he boarded the ferry at Twenty-Sixth Street, to steam towards the men and women he hoped to comfort and save, he had another chance to get it right. He crossed that river as if nothing less than salvation awaited him on the other side. He couldn't wait to get there, and only death would stop him.

THE ALMSHOUSE WAS the third institution to go up on Blackwell's Island, and people who were no longer able to make a living, either through advanced age or infirmity, went there voluntarily. "Misery and destitution brings them in," French would write, and "death sweeps them out."

It would eventually take up about a third of the Island. The two main buildings, one for the men and one for the women, were identical, sitting 650 feet apart from each other in the middle of the Island, opposite Seventieth Street in Manhattan. Between the two main Almshouse buildings was a smaller building which housed the warden and his officers.

The main buildings were three stories high and looked like something out of the French Quarter of New Orleans. Iron staircases led up to embellished, scrolled verandas running along the second and third floors. If it weren't for the location, you'd almost expect to see well-dressed men and women out under parasols, sipping mint juleps. But the Almshouse sat between the Workhouse and the Penitentiary, and that summed up exactly where everyone thought this class of people—the poor and the disabled—belonged, criminals in either direction, three of a kind, all of whom, to one degree or another, deserved punishment. Anyone out on the balconies was most likely there to escape what awaited them inside.

In 1867, two one-story pavilions on the Almshouse grounds that had formerly housed the lunatic overflow from the Asylum were cleaned, repaired, painted, and designated the Hospital for Incurables. "In these buildings are quartered those who are afflicted with incurable diseases, but who require no medical attention." The patients were overseen by one nurse and one orderly, who would get their instructions from the visiting physician who stopped by occasionally to direct their care.

The hospital became a small central core of hopelessness in an already well-established array of despair. A commissioner once acknowledged that if he were put there, "I do not think I could stand it a week." Rev. French would write, "The history of many of these incurables is a tragedy," and they "would make a volume which few could endure to read." Nonetheless, some of the patients attained sideshow-attraction status. One woman, who'd been there eight years, was "the wonder of every visitor," French declared. "She is called the ossified woman, who cannot use her body save to turn her head with a trifling motion. Her hands and arms most visitors can but glance at when uncovered. . . . The strange thing about her is yet to be told. . . . She is the most cheerful person to be seen, meets every one with a smile, never utters a complaint or an impatient word, and is always thankful for the smallest favor. Some Christian soul has sent her a book-holder, which, at her bedside, holds the book that she is reading. Reading is her great enjoyment."

A few months after the Hospital for Incurables became operational, an Asylum for the Indigent Blind was created, although they didn't get their own building. They made do with two wards in the men's Almshouse and two in the women's until 1893, when new pavilions were erected for the Hospital for Incurables. Then, despite being described by the warden as "two antiquated one-story wooden structures, possessing none of the modern sanitary improvements or appliances which are deemed so essential to the well-being of defective and dependent humanity," the indigent blind were moved into the pavilions the incurables had just vacated.

All three establishments, the Almshouse, the Hospital for Incurables, and Asylum for the Indigent Blind, were overseen by the Almshouse warden (although the Hospital for Incurables was to some degree co-managed by Charity Hospital).

In the beginning, the attitude of the commissioners towards the Almshouse inmates appeared warm. In 1848, the year the main buildings were finished, the commissioners wrote that to the people committed there, the Almshouse was "an asylum of happiness in their declining years." That position began to erode almost immediately, and by 1875 their nurturing attitude had completely vanished. An inviting Almshouse was now the very last thing they desired. "Care has been taken not to diminish the terrors of this last resort of poverty, because it has been deemed better that a few should test the minimum rate at which existence can be preserved, than that the many should find the poor house so comfortable a home that they would brave the shame of pauperism to gain admission to it."

With the exception of widows and the permanently disabled, the poor were entirely responsible for their penniless state, and many thought there was a semblance of justice in finding out how little it took to keep them alive. "Poverty," journalist Junius Henri Browne explained in 1869, "is the only crime society cannot forgive."

TO SECURE A spot in the Almshouse, New Yorkers applied for admission at the office of the Superintendent of Outdoor Poor. After 1869, that office was located at 66 Third Avenue, in a two-story building designed by James Renwick and described by the *New York Times* as something that could be mistaken for a "costly looking barn." The setup inside was somewhat similar to police court. The superintendent sat behind a raised platform, but unlike at court, applicants would climb the platform to make their case. Their claims were investigated by a "visitor," who would verify the cause of their destitution. Were they truly disabled, for instance? The visitors would also try to find out if the person had friends or family in a position to help them. If they were found "friendless and penniless," and were residents of New York City, they were sent to the Almshouse.

The goal was to limit admissions to only the truly destitute and those currently incapable of working. In time, as the rules for admission became more and more stringent, for the most part only "the old and decrepit" and people missing one or more arms and legs were admitted, along with the excess inmates from other institutions like the Lunatic Asylum and the Workhouse. When maimed Civil War soldiers started showing up, a Soldiers' Retreat was established in the east wing of the Inebriate Asylum on Wards Island.

Despite the increased restrictions, overcrowding was an ever-present issue. An average of around 2,500 people were received at the Almshouse yearly. Because the Almshouse buildings were designed to accommodate only 600 people each, every night a large number of the most vulnerable and disabled people in New York City ended up huddled on every available square inch of floor space, where they'd lay shivering in the winter, or sweltering in the summer.

In 1882, as Edison was lighting up Manhattan, Mary Williams was moved into the Almshouse from the Workhouse, where she'd been sentenced for vagrancy. Her presence in the Almshouse was highly unusual because the inmates of the Almshouse were almost entirely white, and Mary Williams was a Creek Indian. On the day the census was taken in the Almshouse there were two black men, four black women, and one man who was listed as "brown." (Mary Williams was described as "Red.") Where were all the poor black people in New York City?

They weren't on Blackwell's Island in huge numbers. Each wing of the Workhouse, for instance, had a small separate section for "colored" inmates. The Department of Public Charities and Correction did not list Workhouse inmates by race, but in the 1870 federal census there were 11 black inmates out of a total of 1,360 in the Workhouse that day, and in the 1880 census there were 5 out of 812.

Over in the Lunatic Asylum, in 1871, the last year they supplied numbers by race, 6 men and 13 women were listed as "colored." That amounted to 2.57 percent of the people committed that year. In Charity Hospital, the largest hospital on the island, there were 41 black men and 92 black women, making up 1.7 percent of the people admitted that year. The percentage of blacks sentenced to the Penitentiary that year, however, 91 men and 24 women, came to a little over 6.5 percent. By the beginning of the next century, the percentage of black inmates in the Penitentiary would climb to 12 percent, and it would continue to rise from there.

Race wasn't broken out in all the institutions, however, and one place that didn't list inmates by race was the Almshouse (the figures above came from the federal census). In the beginning, when the Almshouse was part of Bellevue, blacks were housed there along with the whites, although they were segregated. The Common Council was concerned that the Almshouse was luring an "undue proportion of freed Slaves," but an 1837 report paints a picture of such unimaginable cruelty it's hard to see how anyone could seriously believe black people would find life in the Almshouse tempting:

> In the Building assigned to colored subjects, was an exhibition of squalid misery . . . never witnessed by your Commissioners in any public receptacle, for even the most [abandoned] dregs of human society. Here . . . was a scene of neglect, and filth, and putrefaction, and vermin. . . . The same apparel and the same bedding, had been alternately used by the sick, the dying, the convalescent, and those in health, for a long period. . . . It was a scene, the recollections of which are too sickening to describe.

Apparently the Almshouse warden couldn't get rid of black inmates fast enough. In 1818, the Common Council minutes record a "coloured man" from the Almshouse who was put into a coffin while still alive.

In response to this deplorable state of affairs, a group of philanthropists pooled their money and in 1839 created what came to be known as the Colored Home. (The founders included Nancy Jay and her sister, Mrs. Maria Bauyer, both daughters of John Jay, the first chief justice of the New York Supreme Court and the president of the Continental Congress.) The Colored Home began in a house along the Hudson River with only ten inmates, and by 1848 they had settled into a building on Sixty-Fifth Street, just east of First Avenue. The Sixty-Fifth Street home had separate wings for men and women; later they added a hospital, a Lying-in Department for pregnant women, and a nursery. Generally around 600 people or more were admitted and discharged yearly.

The Colored Home rescued the Almshouse commissioners from an awkward and badly managed situation, and in 1845 the managers of the Colored Home and the commissioners entered into a mutually satisfactory arrangement. The commissioners agreed to contribute 60 cents a week toward board and clothing for each Colored Home inmate and the Colored Home agreed to take in all the black and destitute citizens of the city. (In 1866 this was increased to 15 cents a day for regular inmates and 26 cents a day for inmates of the hospital.) The Home received much-needed funds and the commissioners fulfilled their responsibility to care for the poor "colored" people of New York City. The city was getting the better side of the bargain, however. The Board of Aldermen noted that it cost them less to support 297 people in the Colored Home than it did to feed and clothe 177 people in the city prison.

The managers of the Colored Home were not unaware of the discrepancy. Every year Dr. Samuel Whitall, a Quaker and the resident physician of the Colored Home, would write that what they received was less than other institutions which took in and supported the city's poor. "I have so often urged the claims of the Colored Home to a larger revenue than it now receives, that to repeat them at this time may seem both trite and use-less." But each year he would try again. "Until the 'color line' be effectu-ally broken down, and the African race be recognized as entitled to all the rights and privileges of citizenship . . . it has claims upon the benevolent which have heretofore been too much disregarded."

Life for black children in the Bellevue Almshouse was equally bleak. "On visiting the Alms House at Bellevue about this period," the 1851 An-nual Report of the Governors of the Almshouse read, "the colored children were found collected in a cellar, under the care of a man of intemperate habits, who was also at intervals deranged." In the summer of 1837, five children were pulled from that basement and taken to a cottage on Twelfth Street, in an area now known as the West Village in Manhattan. They were among the first inmates in the Colored Orphan Asylum, founded by Quak-ers Anna H. Shotwell, Hannah Shotwell Murray, Hannah's daughter Mary Murray, and others. After a fire in 1842 they moved to a building on Fifth Avenue between Forty-Third and Forty-Fourth Streets.

The Almshouse commissioners were presented with a similar advan-tageous opportunity. Here was an organization willing to take care of the black pauper children of New York City, a group they were ostensibly re-sponsible for, although it took the commissioners almost ten years to ac-knowledge it and respond. In 1845 they agreed to pay 50 cents a week per child, with a cap of one hundred inmates, for a total weekly maximum of $50 (two years later they raised the weekly upper limit to $200). As far as the commissioners were concerned, between the Colored Home and the Colored Orphan Asylum, they'd now satisfied all their obligations to pro-vide aid to the struggling black citizens of New York.

The black community was not initially thrilled with the Orphan Asy-lum. According to Leslie M. Harris in her book, *In the Shadow of Slavery: African Americans in New York City, 1626–1863*, black residents balked at the low expectations the founders originally had for the children, who were essentially being groomed for a life of servitude and menial labor. When money left in a will for the "education and benefit of colored people" was given to the Orphan Asylum, an editorial appeared on December 30, 1837, in the black newspaper, the *Colored American*. While praising the Asylum for its work, the editorial pointed out "it is by no means an institution of learning, but rather a branch of the Almshouse."

Relations with the black community took a turn for the better in 1846 when the Orphan Asylum replaced its white doctors with James McCune Smith, the first black American to receive a medical degree, and a highly respected leader. "McCune Smith's appointment," Harris writes, "signaled the managers' slowly expanding vision of the various roles of which blacks were capable." The quality of the education at the Orphan Asylum gradually improved.

LIKE MARY WILLIAMS, when black adults ended up in the Almshouse instead of the Colored Home, it was usually because they'd started out at the Workhouse and were transferred when the Workhouse ran out of space.

Once they entered the Almshouse, people of color were processed like any other inmates. The admission logbooks recorded their race, age, where they were born, the state of their health, their marital status, whether or not the inmate or their parents where drinkers, the extent of their education, their occupation, and what kind of labor they were capable of, if any. The records would then briefly list what brought the person so low, sometimes saying nothing more than "destitution." Occasionally the descriptions were more vivid, and distinctly sadder, like, "Loss [sic] forepart both arms thrashing machine." Almshouse managers would have to determine if there was any hope of the inmate ever becoming self-supporting again.

When intake was complete, the personal effects of the newly admitted were taken, boxed, and noted in a ledger, to be returned if the inmate was discharged, or given to their surviving family if they died. Many emptied their pockets of ferry tickets they would never use or pawn tickets for items they would never reclaim. Eva Scheinerman, who was admitted on

September 28, 1893, left $7.83 in cash and a package addressed to George F. Britton containing two "pocket-books and a hand bag." Britton was the Secretary of the Department of Public Charities and Correction, and the ledger does not explain why a pauper would leave all her worldly possessions to a Department official. (Britton was later found to have embezzled funds meant for inmates.) "We cannot tell the thousandth part of the sad and sorrowful story," Rev. French wrote, "of the lives of these self-destroyed wrecks or perchance victims of social wrong."

According to the record for Mary Williams, she was fifty-six years old when admitted, and she was born in Savannah, Georgia, the daughter of a chief of the Creek Nation (also known as the Muscogee Nation). She was temperate, could read and write, and her occupation was listed as "housework." The reason for her "Existing Cause of Dependence" was vagrancy, and because vagrancy was a crime, she was originally sentenced to the Workhouse. Her records also indicate that she was made a widow when she was thirty-seven years old and that her husband, sailor William Williams, was killed in a particularly dramatic way. He'd been beaten to death during the infamous New York City draft riots of 1863.

A mob had torn through the city at the height of summer that year in response to a recently enacted draft law. What started out as a reasonable protest against a law that allowed the rich to get out of serving by either finding a substitute or paying $300 devolved into a riot. The protestors were mostly working-class Irish men, but there were also women and children among them. They initially focused on the buildings and draft offices that housed the devices used to call the names of the drafted, and nearby stores (as well as the mayor's home), but as their numbers grew their anger spread to another perceived source of all their troubles, and a much easier target—blacks (and those sympathetic to the black community). Before federal troops managed to quell the riot, over one hundred people, both black and white, were killed, including at least twenty children. One twelve-year-old boy, who probably entered the fray because it was irresistibly exciting, burned to death during a particularly lethal skirmish at the Armory at Second Avenue and Twenty-First Street.

Early in the morning on the second day of the riot, the black sailor William Williams left his ship, the U.S. transport *Belvidere*, and had the misfortune of crossing paths with a drunken Irish laborer named Edward Canfield. Williams had stopped at the corner of Leroy and Washington Streets in the West Village to ask an eleven-year-old boy named Edward Ray where he might find a grocery store. Canfield was just exiting a liquor store, presumably storing up on what he saw as essential riot fortification. While the boy watched, Canfield knocked Williams down then jumped on top of him and started beating him. Then he leaned on the shoulder of a man who stood next to him and kicked out Williams's eyes with the toes of his boots.

Men and boys who were already out and about and looking for trouble gathered. As neighbors watched from their windows, Canfield and others continued to beat and kick Williams. Emma Flandrow later testified that when she first started watching, Williams was half sitting up, raised up on one elbow, but the growing crowd battered him all the way down. Her next-door neighbor James Lamb, she noticed, had come out to join the murderers. Flandrow saw him take off his coat, hand it to an onlooker, and then push up his shirt sleeves and look around for a weapon. A nearby flagstone caught his eye. In seconds he was slamming it down on Williams's chest, breaking ribs. While Flandrow and others watched the "show," another man came by and tried to stab Williams, but "he could not get it in," according to the boy Edward Ray.

In all the pages of testimony there is no record of Williams having ever called out for help. Perhaps because he knew there was there no help to be had, and crying out would have only inflamed his attackers. When the killers were done, "there were several cheers given," and a call for "vengeance on every nigger in New York," as most of them moved on to look for other victims. Canfield went back to the liquor store, now blood-spattered.

Margaret Holmes, who had also been watching from a window, left her apartment to enter the circle of remaining men, women, and children who stood around, staring at Williams, who was still alive and now trying, but unable, to speak. Two bystanders finally ran to the station house on Greenwich Street. The police carted Williams off to New York Hospital where he died two hours later.

During the riot, black children were also considered acceptable candidates for murder. On July 13, the day before Williams was killed, several thousand men, women, and children made their way to the now thriving Colored Orphan Asylum. It was around 4 p.m. and the mob had just burnt down the Bull's Head Hotel on Forty-Fourth Street. The Asylum managers had been alerted to the mob's intentions just minutes before and all the children and their caretakers were huddled in the room used for assemblies. When the mob broke down the front door with an axe, the superintendent and matron led 233 children out through the back piazza.

Many years later one of the orphans, Thomas Barnes, who was fourteen years old at the time of the riot, wrote about his experiences that day. He and his brother and three other children had bolted as soon as the mob reached the front gates. Everywhere they ran they were stopped by the sight of angry crowds. They were headed for a church on Forty-First Street when concerned residents told them to find another direction. They looked down the block. "We could see a colored man hanging from a lamppost." They were eventually spotted by a policeman and two firemen who got them to the station house at Thirty-Fifth Street, where they joined their classmates, their superintendent, their matron, and others. Although the Colored Orphan Asylum had been pillaged and burned, no one was killed in the encounter except a bystander, a ten-year-old white child named Jane Barry, who was watching from the street and was crushed by a bureau the rioters had thrown out of the windows of the orphanage.

At the station house the 233 children were put in the basement in "ten small cells, five on either side of a hall," which normally held one prisoner each. With so many children crowding the cells there was no room to sit or lie down, and they were forced to remain like that for the next twenty-four hours until they were moved within the building. The other prisoners, incarcerated rioters, tried to hit the children through the bars. When that failed they came up with an ingenious method of tormenting the exhausted and terrified children. Every cell had a faucet and a sink. The rioters "let the water run on the floor, compelling us to stand in the filthy water from their cells," making an already wretched situation that much more miserable.

The children and the Asylum managers remained at the station house for eighty hours while plans were made to get them out of the mob's reach and onto Blackwell's Island. On the third morning they were led up and out into the street. Twenty policemen were stationed in the front of the group and twenty more waited to bring up the rear. Flanking their position were fifty "Zouaves with their glittering bayonets on either side," each man more than ready to take on anyone who got in his way. (The Zouaves were an elite volunteer regiment in the army, known for their dashing uniforms.) The order was given and the children marched down the street two-by-two between the lines of soldiers. The crowds were in "awe of the determined aspect of those soldiers." No one dared make a move. The decks of the ship that would take them to the Island had been cleared and cannons installed, now aimed at the still volatile crowds.

More cannons lined the shores of Blackwell's Island, arranged for by Almshouse Warden Nehemiah P. Anderson, who ordered his men "to shoot the first suspicious boat." Anderson welcomed the children and made sure they were immediately fed and dressed in fresh, clean clothes (they were still wearing what they'd put on for classes days earlier and continued to wear throughout their stay in the filthy jail cells). Boatloads of refugees continued to arrive throughout the day. There weren't enough beds for everyone, but the children didn't care. They took up every available inch on the lovely wrought-iron balconies that wrapped around the second and third floors, and they stretched out on every staircase step. The weather was sweltering that July, and sleeping outside was not only a relief, it was an adventure, like camping out.

The children were grateful to Anderson, who was exceedingly kind to them, and who often invited them into his home for dinner. But they were head over heels for the swashbuckling engineer Elijah T. Simpson, who "always carried a brace of revolvers and a whip in his belt," and who "made life happy for us." (The Almshouse engineer looked after the buildings, plumbing, the gas fittings, and roads.) Simpson organized games and other activities for the children, and while he did everything in his power to make their "stay on the island a holiday in every sense," sixty years later Barnes still remembered that he could be "cruel in the extreme to the paupers and men under him." (Barnes did not provide an example, but perhaps it involved the whip).

Anderson meanwhile provided space so that the children's schooling continued. Barnes recalled a different and unintended education. "We saw the criminal at close range in the penitentiary and workhouse. . . . We saw the almshouse filled with hundreds of paupers, mostly old and decrepit . . . . We saw insane . . . exhibiting every phase of mental derangement. . . . Oh, what a sight! What a lesson we learned from their afflictions."

While the children managed to avoid harm from thousands of drunk and angry rioters bent on their destruction, they couldn't escape all the dangers of Blackwell's Island. Two boys who'd unwisely decided to go swimming "were carried out to sea, and we never saw or heard from them" again.

Later, the commissioners of the Department of Public Charities and Correction would complain that after having taken in over 200 children and housing and feeding them for 105 days, they could find "no allusion whatever made to this Department" in the Colored Orphan Asylum's annual report. Instead, the Asylum managers "seem at all times willing to avoid the stamp of Alms house reputation."

Although the managers of the Colored Orphan Asylum had expressed gratitude, the truth is the Almshouse had a terrible reputation when it came to the care of children. It's not inconceivable that the Asylum managers may have wanted to downplay any connection. The same year the children of the Colored Orphan Asylum had been taken in, the commissioners of the Department of Public Charities and Correction wrote, "Our most startling account of loss of life is to be found in our statistics of the children at the Alms House." While Blackwell's Island wasn't a healthy place for anyone, it was positively lethal for children. Mortality rates for abandoned infants frequently rose to over 80 percent. "It would be an act of humanity," one superintendent conceded, "if each foundling were given a fatal dose of opium on its arrival." One physician "was shown one miserable infant which was regarded as a prodigy because it had managed to attain the age of two months."

The children at the Colored Orphan Asylum received much better care than the pauper children who ended up in the Almshouse. Of the 954 children in the Almshouse in 1865, 580 died, or just under 61 percent. At the Colored Orphan Asylum, 11 of the 283 children died, or just under 4 percent.

In their defense, the Almshouse was responsible for a lot more children, many of whom had arrived in the worst possible condition. In the nineteenth century, swarms of these children roamed the city in packs. Their numbers are hard to pin down, but estimates made during the worst years ranged from 5,000 to 50,000. "Street children," they were called, or "gutter snipes." It's almost impossible to imagine, yet thousands of children lived and died in those gutters and people strolled right by them the way we walk by homeless adults today. The foundlings who arrived at the Almshouse were, according to the commissioners, "often brought from the subterranean holes of our worst locations, by the most wretched of mothers in human form, with sunken eyes, emaciated limbs, and filthy remnants of miserable wrappings. Strangers to light, to comfort or to home, the all but lifeless form is brought forth, its little life blighted at its birth, and poisoned by the horrid distillations dealt out to its vagrant mother—and thus it comes to us. Is it surprising that a merciful Providence spares so few of these unfortunate offspring?"

In 1866, steps were finally taken to bring mortality rates down. Previously, the Almshouse accepted infants and children up to fifteen years old, although many older children were sent to the nursery department on Randalls Island. The commissioners now decided that infants and healthy children over the age of two would no longer be sent to the Almshouse. An Infants' Bureau was established and plans were approved for a new infants' hospital that would be built on Randalls Island. The hospital started accepting patients in 1869, but mortality rates for foundlings were ultimately high there as well. Sick children were still admitted to Charity Hospital on Blackwell's, and in large numbers, but many were also sent to Nursery Hospital on Randalls Island. Meanwhile, other institutions like the Foundling Asylum of the Sisters of Charity arose (later known as the New York Foundling Hospital, now called New York Foundling).

In time, except for those born at the maternity hospital, which started accepting patients in 1878, and those who were still being sent to Charity Hospital, caring for children on Blackwell's was slowly phased out. Criminal children (juvenile delinquents) were already being sentenced to the House of Refuge on Randalls Island, although small numbers of children from ten to fifteen years old continued to be sentenced to the Penitentiary, and women with very young children and infants were sometimes allowed to bring their babies with them when they were sentenced to the Workhouse. The rest were placed in homes, foster homes, and various private and religious institutions.

The Children's Law would pass in 1875, removing any remaining children between the ages of three (later lowered to two) and sixteen from the Almshouse (and all poorhouses). However, a handful of children between ten and fifteen years old were still housed in the Almshouse depending on special circumstances, the whims of the Almshouse managers at the time, and space. Some officials even wanted to keep the children in the

Almshouse. A few years after the 1875 law went into effect, Josephine Shaw Lowell (who was instrumental in helping pass the law) would be shocked how "even now, incredible as it may appear, there are men in the State . . . who are ready to condemn helpless children to a lifelong pauperism by repealing the law of 1875, and to rear them in poorhouses, simply because it costs 'the county' a few cents more a day to give them such a home as will save them from that misery."

The Children's Law did not cover penal institutions, and justices continued to send children to the Penitentiary and the Workhouse.

IN THE YEARS that Rev. French was ministering to the people in the Almshouse, the average daily population went from around 1,000 to over 2,500 men and women who were living out the remainder of their lives there, as if buried alive. French wrote in his 1882 annual report, "The life—a dull routine of eating and sleeping, untouched by the stir and excitement of the world without, unmoved by its emulations and ambitions— tends to degrade and brutalize."

In reality, they were just barely eating. While intake workers would write down "destitution" as their reason for coming to the Almshouse, French wrote in his annual report that they were "destitute of daily food." He opined, "In vain is any effectual ministry to the soul," when "you give them not those things that are needful to the body." Even though they were feeding the inmates at a rate of 7 cents a day, a former commissioner complained "that the poor-house people were too well fed. They ought to be cut down to the lowest limit." What could be lower than what a *New York Times* reporter found when he lifted the cloth covering the inmate's meat, which he described as something you'd find on the "field amputating-table after one of Grant's battles. It was hideous, covered with dirt, blue, bruised," and "reeking with nameless corruptions."

Like the Workhouse inmates, the Almshouse inmates who fell ill were treated in an in-house hospital instead of being sent to Charity Hospital. For them, there was now little hope that they'd ever see anything other than the inside of the Almshouse again. The issue wasn't keeping them away from the innocent poor, as it was with the Workhouse patients. The commissioners insisted that the care the Almshouse inmates received would be better, and that they were sparing "these old people from the dangers and discomforts of a transfer to Charity Hospital, when, perhaps, within a few hours of death." French would later say that the Almshouse was made the receptacle of anyone close to death in order to lower the mortality rates of the other institutions. There was no running water, hot, cold, or otherwise, anywhere in the Almshouse. The only way to even get to the second and third floors, where the hospital wards were located, was from the outside, via the stairs and the balconies. For a proper bath they'd have to go back out onto the balcony and climb down the stairs to the cellar, where water was brought in (later, to separate bathhouses). There were, of course, no bathrooms.

While on his daily visits to the wards, French was sometimes the first to discover when a patient had died. In 1897, Homer Folks, who at the time was Secretary of the State Charities Aid Association of New York, described a tragicomic scene at the Almshouse hospital which illustrates how this could happen. "When the visitors inquired for the person in charge, there was considerable confusion and loud calls for, we will say, 'Billy,' who soon came tottering down from the upper end of the ward, a picture of confusion and incompetency. This one old man, who might more properly have been a patient, had sole charge of these sixty sick people. It was a hot day in mid-summer. One poor old man who had pulled down the mosquito-netting from over his face, and was too weak to replace it, was being tortured by flies. The visitor asked the orderly if this man were not in a dying condition. The orderly, who until that time had been paying no attention to the patient, looked at him and said he 'guessed he was,' but did nothing further for him. The patient died later that afternoon."

French once found an eighty-three-year-old blind man shivering in his room. As in all the institutions, inmates' clothes were taken away and replaced with inferior items, which often lead to pneumonia and consumption. "They took away my overcoat . . . and my flannel undershirt and drawers," the blind man said, "and I am very cold. That north door is opened continually, and the draft is freezing me." The windows and doors were kept open due to the stench of unwashed bodies. When a visitor asked about the smell in the women's Almshouse, and the fact that it was very cold on the men's side, a commissioner whispered "Women are always less cleanly than men," not mentioning that they had few resources to get clean. It was colder on the men's side, he said, because they could stand the breeze from the open windows that the women could not.

But could they? The only heat in the Almshouse was provided by coal stoves, one to a ward. These may have managed to keep the small area around the stove warm, but it would not have reached all the rooms on the ward. The old man without a coat had no choice but to just sit there, for "days and weeks, in his blindness; very infirm," French wrote, and he "could not get about without aid," which, in any case, "was not rendered him." There was no one except French to occasionally bring him closer to their one meager source of warmth. "I regard the Alms House as the tide-table to mark how high the waters of Life are flowing through the hearts of the children of God." The tides were perpetually low. The shivering man he had come upon soon died.

Another priest on the Island included French in his own annual report one year. "A poor cripple . . . hobbling along on two sticks, bent double with rheumatism . . . asked to see the Rev. Mr. French, to whom he told his sorrowful tale of pain and suffering. The venerable priest . . . at once procured from his scant store a pair of warm woolen stockings." French never stopped trying to make up for the deficit of care out of his own pocket. "Just at that moment I was called away," the priest continued, "and when I returned I saw the good old man, with his silver locks, bending down and putting these stockings on the poor fellow, who could not do it for himself." The Almshouse man, who had not expected this response, only

a sympathetic ear, was sobbing. The priest who was watching had to hold
back tears as well. After years without proper food or clothes, a simple pair
of socks can decimate the defenses of a battle-scarred pauper and a sea-
soned observer.

Dr. William G. Le Boutillier would later resign from the Medical Board
of Visitors to the Charitable Institutions of the City due the number of pre-
ventable deaths in the Almshouse. In a letter to the editor of the *New York
Times* he wrote that when travelers to the Island strayed "from the path
prepared to give the visiting public the best impression" they walked into
scenes that defy "the dictates of humanity and the ordinary laws of health."
The Board's calls for more food, clothing and the practice of basic hygiene were ignored while the commissioners continued to focus on bringing costs down. This resulted in rising deaths even as the total number of
inmates declined. "The weakness of any attempts at reform on the part
of the Medical Board becomes clear when it is known that its members are
appointed by the Commissioners of Charities and Correction, and that
the appointments are made partly through political 'influence.'" Such was
the case, of course, everywhere on Blackwell's and just like staff at the
other institutions, the physicians on the Island were reluctant to complain
too loudly, he wrote, because they didn't want to lose their position. Le
Boutillier's letter to the editor was his last-ditch attempt to effect change
by appealing to the general public.

French was particularly concerned and appalled about the number
of widows who were routinely dumped at the Almshouse. He repeatedly
railed against their abandonment, perhaps hoping his objections might
make their way into Sunday sermons throughout the city. It offended his
sense of duty, the way they were brought there "to wear out a miserable existence, in a place where they are brought into daily contact with the large
proportion of vicious and degraded people necessarily admitted to a public
Alms-House." Even the wealthy "pack off their widows to this institution
to be 'herded,' until they are discharged by the Warden or by death."

Death, of course, was the issue. For many, this would be their only way out, and the inmates were painfully aware of it. "I am dying," one inmate said to French when he came to administer Holy Communion. "I shall never get over this." Another woman "kept her shroud ready" for that inevitable day, and she didn't "want people to know that I have a shroud in my trunk ready for me when I die," she told French. "I hope it will not be stolen."

If the afflictions associated with old age didn't carry the inmates off, they were usually done in by tuberculosis or diarrhea, two of the leading causes of death in the Almshouse. They might also end up murdered by a fellow inmate who really belonged in the Lunatic Asylum. As the city recovered from the draft riots in 1863, Anne O'Neil, an eighty-year-old Irish woman, was murdered by Margaret Finn, identified only as a "crazy woman."

Almshouse inmates were also vulnerable to the occasional, and deadly, cholera or typhus outbreak. On January 2, 1893, for the first time in twenty years, trips between the city and Blackwell's Island ceased. Almshouse inmate Kate Anderson, who'd started showing symptoms of typhus, had just been transferred to Riverside Hospital, a hospital for infectious diseases that moved from Blackwell's to North Brother Island in 1885. (North Brother Island is famous as the place where Typhoid Mary was confined.)

Before antibiotics were developed, typhus would spread rapidly, especially in places like the Almshouse, where all the factors that increase the chances for a typhus epidemic were present: over-crowding, filth, cold, and hunger. (It was later discovered that typhus comes from a bacteria transmitted by lice and fleas.) Typhus was also particularly lethal for the elderly, and Kate Anderson had potentially come into contact with an estimated 1,000 to 1,200 old women.

Anderson died within hours of her arrival on North Brother Island. When French showed up at the dock the next day, he was told that if he crossed over to Blackwell's Island he would not be permitted to return to Manhattan and his family. French climbed aboard anyway. He conducted services at both the Almshouse and the Lunatic Asylum, just as he always

did, and, contrary to what he'd been told, he was allowed to take a boat
back home. After that, he came from and went to the Island freely, but until
the quarantine was lifted he was barred from reentering the Almshouse.

Despite the fears of an outbreak, police justices and the Superintendent
of Outdoor Poor continued to send people to the Island. The situation was
made even more perilous by the decision to not allow convicts or inmates
to leave. As "the stream of corruption of body, soul and spirit continued to
pour in," French related, eighty men who'd finished their sentences were
not released, creating a human pile-up of pent-up fear and tension, and
the possibility of a revolt. As storms of rain and snow raged, anyone suspected of having been infected was hustled into hastily erected tents. Given
the level of panic, the inside of those tents must have been pandemonium,
French later wrote. In the end, only a small number of people actually died
from the disease. Many more succumbed to tuberculosis.

That same year, "an old German, working year after year in the tailor's
shop, without recompense, poorly clad and poorly fed, at last grew tired of
life," French wrote. After supper one night in the Almshouse, the man met
with an old friend, a fellow inmate, and together they "talked of their common miseries." The old man then emptied his pockets and gave his friend
"three pennies, all his store," saying, "I have no further use for them." It
was early evening when they parted. The friend went back to his ward, and
the old German "walked out to the wall on the bank of the river, jumped
in and was not missed until the morning."

French did what he could for the inmates, often reaching out to estranged relatives. Once, he tried writing to the sister of a woman who'd
been a prostitute and who was now blind. The inmate was haunted by the
idea that she was being punished for the life she led. "I cannot see; but I
think all day long." The sister never answered and the woman died alone.
"She met with no mercy at the hand of an only sister" to whom he'd written in vain.

Dying was frightening enough to contemplate, but there were two
things about losing their lives in the Almshouse that even those who

welcomed death as a release dreaded. They were summed up by one man when he rejected French's overture to embrace Christianity. "In what respect is it worth while to be a Christian, if, after this life of misery here, I must be cut up and buried like a dead dog; and Christians, who profess to be my brethren, do not care enough for me to give me a decent burial. I am poor, but I have never been a criminal."

The old men and women were right to shrink from some of the boats piled with bodies approaching Blackwell's. Everyone in the Almshouse knew that dissection and the potter's field was their likely fate. It was all perfectly legal. It began with an act in 1789 which gave the court the power to have the bodies of those who'd been sentenced to death delivered to physicians and medical students for dissection. Not long after the act passed the number of crimes which could result in an execution was reduced. To address the shortfall, an 1854 "act to promote medical science" was crafted by legislators, which allowed the wardens of the prisons, penitentiaries, and almshouses to similarly hand over the unclaimed remains of paupers. The pool of available bodies increased, outraging groups like the Irish Emigrant Aid Society, whose dead would make up most of those scientific contributions.

One of the few conditions placed on the recipients of the bodies was a proper burial of the remains when they were done. This translated to internment in the potter's field, which was on Wards Island at the time of the 1854 law. In 1869 the site of the potter's field was moved to Hart Island, a small island north of Blackwell's, off the shores of the Bronx.

The ritual that followed a death in the Almshouse became depressingly and inexorably routine. "The old hand-dray of years past," French wrote in his annual report, "still carries the bodies to the filthy dead-house for dissection [or elsewhere]; and thence to the dock; thence by boat to the Morgue, and the Potter's Field on Hart's Island."

There was one aspect about this practice that especially outraged French as a Christian. "It is not surprising that even the unbelieving inmates who look forward to death should have a horror of the surgeon's knife, and the Potter's Field," French wrote. But for those "who believe their bodies to be The Temples of the Holy Ghost," it was sacrilegious. "Are not the bodies of her dead poor of the same value in the Lord's sight, as the bodies of the rich? Why not bury them in her consecrated ground? Why a pauper burial?"

A pauper burial consisted of being piled into one of the group trenches dug out by workers at an institution called the Industrial School. After purchasing Hart Island in 1868, the city promptly handed it over to the Department of Public Charities and Correction. In addition to selecting it as the new site for the city's potter's field (officially called the City Cemetery) the Department also built another asylum for the insane there, along with various hospitals, and what they called an Industrial School. The Industrial School was essentially a penal institution for boys, but it was intended as a gentler alternative to the House of Refuge, a detention center that was created in order to separate younger criminals from adults. "To the Industrial School on Hart's Island are committed vagrant boys too old to be sent to the Nurseries on Randall's Island, habitual truants from school and incorrigible boys," the Department of Public Charities and Correction's 1870 annual report reads. "It is really a branch work-house for the younger inmates," a later president of the Department of Public Charities and Correction characterized it. In 1876 it officially became the Branch Workhouse, and by the next year there were no longer any boys there, only men and women.

The task of digging out the trenches initially fell to men from the Workhouse who'd been assigned to the Industrial School (the annual reports are vague about whether or not the boys helped), and later by inmates of the Branch Workhouse. (Today the work is done by inmates of Rikers.) When the trenches were ready, workers would stack 150 men and women into each trench assigned to the adults, and a thousand infants and more (sometimes many more) into the trenches designated for babies. The number of dead babies usually surpassed the number of adults. In 1871, for instance, 2,243 infants up to the age of one were buried on Hart Island, nearly twice the number of adults that year.

The city allowed bodies to be disinterred as long as it was within a certain time period after burial (today it is nine years). Almshouse inmates were tormented by the possibility "that their bodies might be at the bottom, and dozens laid over them, and so out of reach of all recognition if friends should wish to remove them." After twenty-five years each of the trenches was reused.

The City Cemetery and the Industrial School (and later the Branch Workhouse) were all overseen by none other than Lawrence Dunphy, the man who would go on to replace Rev. Stocking at the Workhouse on Blackwell's Island. Dunphy had been managing the City Cemetery since 1866 (he was a keeper at the Penitentiary before that), and he would continue to manage the cemetery until his transfer to Blackwell's. Perhaps piling untold thousands of poor men, women, and their children into trenches for over twenty years helped mold the strict disciplinarian who came to run the Workhouse on Blackwell's Island.

But Dunphy was also a man of quiet compassion. Hart Island was an abandoned military facility when he got there, with deserted, mussel-strewn beaches and few trees. The lack of trees meant more wind, and gale-force currents would occasionally sweep unimpeded across the trench-filled fields, giving an already desolate place a more fiercely barren feel. So Dunphy planted trees. When a plot was set aside for the internment of soldiers only, Dunphy arranged for head boards which noted the name, age, and date of death for each soldier.

Everyone else was laid underneath white group markers, with only a trench number to indicate their location. No one wanted to end up there. "It is pitiful to hear their prayers for a Christian burial," French wrote. The Guild of St. Elizabeth was established in 1876 to help. At the cost of $11 per burial, for which they were always soliciting funds, the Guild provided burial robes, a coffin, and transportation to St. Michael's Cemetery in Astoria, which had an area specifically designated for the poor. (The Hebrew Free Burial Society was likewise founded to arrange for the burial of paupers of the Jewish faith; however, only six of the 208 people they buried in 1874, for instance, came from Blackwell's Island.)

Every year, anywhere from two to more than four thousand people were buried on Hart Island, and the Guild couldn't provide alternatives for them all. Most of the people at the Almshouse would continue to find their way into a trench, leading French to lament, "The burials of the Alms House dead is a sad business, at best."

It got a little better in 1888. When French first began his mission in 1872, the Almshouse managers would not permit him to conduct services in the Chapel. Eventually he was allowed to hold one Sunday service a month and a service every Thursday. On holidays like Christmas and Easter he had to get special permission. "Until we can have Chapels where our people can worship," French fumed, "at any and all times, without the necessity of 'getting out of the way' for others, who practically claim and use the Chapel for their own, no successful, effectual work can be done." The Catholics did indeed think of the Almshouse chapel as their own. One Jesuit missionary referred to it in a letter as "our chapel at the Alms-House. . . . We have there three neat altars which can be shut up from view by folding doors, for the hall is also used by Protestants." Given that their flock made up most of the inmates of the Almshouse, and everywhere else on the Island, their proprietary feeling is not completely out of line.

Years later a wealthy Episcopalian named George Bliss came to the rescue. Bliss hired architect Frederick Clarke Withers to design the Chapel of the Good Shepherd, which was completed and donated to the New York Protestant City Mission and the inmates of the Almshouse in 1889. (Ironically, Withers was also responsible for the design of the Jefferson Market Courthouse, one of the police courts from which so many people were sent to Blackwell's Island in the first place.)

The chapel offered French validation of his work that was frequent and ongoing. It wasn't just French's ability to freely call the inmates to service *every day* with the "sweet-toned bell" that had been installed in the tower. The chapel also had a large reading room in the basement, something French had been trying to arrange for the Almshouse inmates since he got there. The reading room was open to everyone in the Almshouse, just as he'd always intended. At last they had a place to go outside of the Almshouse, a place that was not only a source of solace and beauty, but of enrichment and stimulation. Whenever French had a day that made him doubt himself and all humanity, he could simply walk over and witness the chapel's salutary effects. For the Protestant inmates, the most meaningful and comforting dimension of Bliss's gift was knowing that before they were laid to rest, wherever that might be, they would at least have a Christian service first, in a chapel built especially for them. For French, it was knowing that, for however many years he had left himself, he would be the one to see them off, in a place that finally treated them as what they were: worthy.

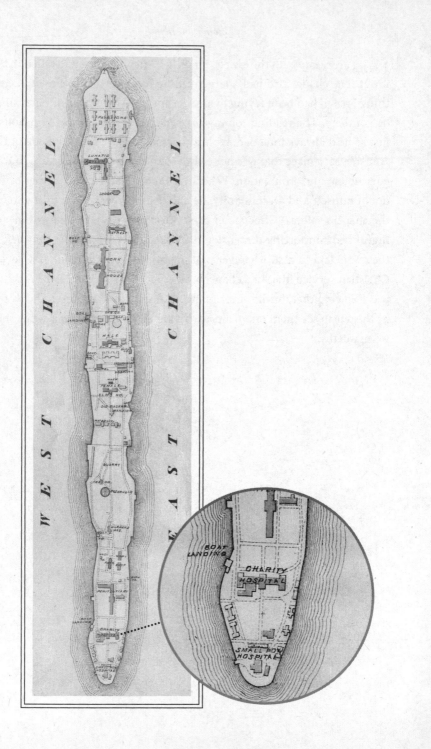

❧ IV ❧

THE HOSPITALS FOR THE POOR

———◆———

IN OPERATION BEGINNING 1832, TO SERVE THE SICK
PEOPLE OF NEW YORK CITY, AND THE INMATES OF THE
PENITENTIARY, WORKHOUSE, AND ALMSHOUSE

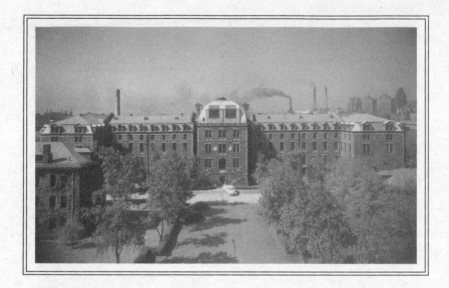

PENITENTIARY HOSPITAL AKA
ISLAND HOSPITAL AKA CHARITY HOSPITAL
AKA CITY HOSPITAL

———◆———

I T STARTED OUT as the Penitentiary Hospital, but it wasn't an actual hospital. It was a room on the top floor of the Penitentiary, and it eventually took over the whole floor. Hundreds of men, most of them suffering from various stages of syphilis, from initial genital ulcers to large and putrid abscesses all over their bodies, were packed into one barred room, without access to a bathroom. Years later it hadn't improved. "I defy the stoutest-hearted layman to go through the wards of this hospital," a *New York Times* reporter wrote, "without fairly growing sick at the stomach."

The women had it better. They were housed in two pavilions at the southern tip of the Island. According to the commissioner overseeing the institution, the location had the "advantage of good air, affording a very necessary element in the cure of the almost *special* disease here treated." Syphilis had no truly effective treatment at the time, but that didn't stop the commissioner from proudly proclaiming in 1847 that "the Penitentiary Hospital is *the* Venereal Hospital of the City" (italics, in both cases, his). It was also, for the poor, the only venereal hospital in the city, and in order to be treated there you had to go to prison first.

Like the Almshouse, the process began at the office of the Superintendent of Outdoor Poor. If sick people couldn't afford a private hospital they would fill out an application to receive medical care at the city hospital, which in the early history of New York meant Bellevue. While they were examined by a physician, someone else was making sure the applicant was truly destitute, with no friends or family who could pay their bills. If everything checked out, they were admitted, but if they had syphilis or another venereal disease, they were turned away and sent instead to police court. The only way for them to get treatment, such as it was before the discovery of antibiotics, was to voluntarily commit themselves to the Penitentiary for vagrancy, where they would eventually be transferred to the top floor.

The new prisoners/patients had to wear prison stripes, and were treated like any other convict at the Penitentiary. Even though they'd committed themselves, the length of their sentence, usually one to six months, was assigned at the whim of the police justice.

Dr. William W. Sanger, who was put in charge of the hospital in 1846, objected. Not everyone who gets syphilis is a criminal, he argued. "A poor woman, without crime or fault on her own part," could contract syphilis from a drunken, philandering husband. A laborer who'd never committed a crime in his life might get drunk one night and catch the disease from a prostitute. "When he comes out of the Hospital, where he has been associated 'with thieves, felons, and murderers,' his self-respect is gone, and he cannot again obtain respectable employment, for he has been in the Penitentiary. Now who is responsible for this man's ruin, and the ruin of his family?"

There were no exceptions. Even children had to go to jail before they could receive care. Sanger's colleague Dr. William Kelly found a girl "not yet 13" being treated for syphilis in the Penitentiary Hospital. If grown women had few opportunities in the nineteenth century, it was even worse for young girls who had to fend for themselves, or help their families. Diarist George Templeton Strong wrote, "No one can walk the length of Broadway without meeting some hideous troop of ragged girls, from twelve years old down, brutalized already almost beyond redemption by premature vice, clad in filthy refuse of the ragpicker's collections, obscene of speech, the stamp of childhood gone from their faces, hurrying along with harsh laughter and foulness on their lips."

In the 1886 book, *Danger! A True History of a Great City's Wiles and Temptations*, the authors, two lawyers who often represented the people they describe, write, "Girls can only sell papers, flowers or themselves, but boys can black boots, sell papers, run errands, carry bundles, sweep out saloons." Young girls were sometimes kidnapped, brought to a disorderly house, then drugged and raped. "I see no wisdom, to say nothing of justice," Kelly railed, "in the law, ordinance, or custom that requires a girl affected with syphilis to become a prisoner before she can become a patient."

Joseph Keen, the warden of the Penitentiary, was one of many who complained that this system only kept the prostitution industry going. Humanity demanded that they treat the afflicted. But once they'd received free medical care, nursing, food, and a warm bed "at the expense of virtuous and laborious tax-payers," the people "who live on the ruin of her soul and body, hasten her return to her city haunts . . . and thus the scene alternates between the house of infamy and the Hospital, until death steps in, and at least relieves the city treasury from any farther [sic] expense than that of a pine coffin, and its transportation to Potter's Field."

The City wanted to get a sense of just how big a problem they had on their hands. How many people suffer from syphilis, Sanger was asked, and what can we do to eradicate this scourge?

In order to address the problem, he told them, they needed more information, and something beyond the kind of statistics that had already been gathered many times before. With the commissioner's blessing, Sanger organized and oversaw a survey of 2,000 prostitutes aged fifteen to seventy-seven. Police trained by Sanger in questioning techniques conducted the actual interviews, and out of this effort came the exhaustive *History of Prostitution*, which was published in 1858.

In answer to the original question *how many cases of syphilis are there out there?*, two fifths of the women interviewed confessed to having had a venereal disease one or more times, although Sanger believed the real number was unquestionably higher. To get a better handle on the total number of cases, it was important to know the number of working prostitutes. While one of the accepted figures cited at the time was 10,000, and others went as high as 30,000 and 50,000, Sanger put it at 7,860. Given that there were more customers than prostitutes, and some of the men became infected and passed the disease on to other prostitutes, not to mention their wives and their future unborn children, that was a lot of potential exposure. Allowing that many cases were not recorded, and others were being treated privately, Sanger estimated that 74,000 cases of venereal disease were being treated every year. (The treatment at the time was mercury, whose side effects include death.) That figure included people who were being treated repeatedly, like syphilitic rounders.

Sanger also confirmed that the child "not yet 13" found by Dr. Kelly was not an isolated occurrence. Of the 6,849 cases of syphilis at the Penitentiary Hospital between 1854 and 1857, 282 of the patients were girls under sixteen. The number rose to 2,285 when young women up to twenty years old were counted. The statistics became downright ghastly when Sanger examined the records for the nursery hospital on Randalls Island. Fifty percent of the children there were being treated for syphilis. The breakdown of those who had contracted the disease in utero from their mothers and those who were infected through sexual contact, the resident physician told him, "can not be stated with accuracy."

Among the many revelations that stand out from Sanger's research is the compassion (and paternalism) he felt towards the prostitutes in his survey. "Their hearts throb with the same sympathies that move the more favored of their sex," he wrote, before describing the arc of their careers with heartbreaking, and unflinching, precision. "Take, for example, the career of a female who enters a house of prostitution at sixteen years of age. Her step is elastic, her eye bright, she is the 'observed of all observers.'" But this period of admiration and prosperity didn't last long. The average prostitute got four good years before it all began to go downhill. "Her physical powers wane under the trials imposed upon them, and her career in a fashionable house of prostitution comes to an end; she must descend in the ladder of vice. . . . To-night you may see her glittering at one of the fashionable theatres; to-morrow she will be found in some one of the infamous resorts which abound in the lower part of the city. . . . To-day she has servants to do her bidding; to-morrow she may be buried in a pauper's coffin and a nameless grave. . . . There is a well understood gradation in this life, and as soon as a woman ceases to be attractive in the higher walks, as soon as her youth and beauty fade, she must either descend in the scale or starve."

Society offered them little chance at redemption, they would discover. "As the last spark of inherent virtue flickers and dies in her bosom, and she becomes sensible that she is indeed lost, that her anticipated happiness proves but splendid misery, she also becomes conscious that the door of reformation is practically closed against her."

"They are, in every sense of the word, outcasts; compelled . . . to eke out a wretched existence by stealing or begging; frequently so miserable that they gladly hail the day on which they are returned to prison."

What was probably the most revealing and surprising, both for the time period and for Sanger, was the response to this question: "What was the cause of your becoming a prostitute?"

Causes	Numbers
Inclination	513
Destitution	525
Seduced and abandoned	258
Drink, and the desire to drink	181
Ill-treatment of parents, relatives, or husbands	164
As an easy life	124
Bad company	84
Persuaded by prostitutes	71
Too idle to work	29
Violated	27
Seduced on board emigrant ships	16
Seduced in emigrant boarding houses	8
Total	2,000

Sanger was shocked by the large number of women who answered *Inclination*, "which can only be understood as meaning a voluntary resort to prostitution in order to gratify the sexual passions. . . . The force of desire can neither be denied nor disputed, but still in the bosoms of most females that force exists in a slumbering state until aroused by some outside influences."

Sanger grasped for reasons to explain feminine lust as a perversion, because to suggest otherwise "would imply innate depravity, a want of true womanly feeling, which is actually incredible." Perhaps regular contact with women "who have yielded to its power," would awaken such desires. Or alcohol. "But it must be repeated, and most decidedly, that without these or some other equally stimulating cause, the full force of sexual desire is seldom known to a virtuous woman." Unlike man, who "is the aggressive animal, so far as sexual desire is involved. Were it otherwise, and the passions in both sexes equal, illegitimacy and prostitution would be far more rife in our midst than at present."

Sanger ended his report with a plea to decriminalize prostitution and to instead "place prostitutes and prostitution under the surveillance of a medical bureau in the Police Department," where they would be subject to medical regulations and mandatory hospitalization, if they were found to be infected.

Sanger had initially resigned in 1847, but he returned in 1853. Between his two stints, he was able to accomplish some measure of reform. He hired assistant resident physicians who lived on the island and who could therefore respond more quickly when needed. He added an apothecary to manage and dispense medications and to keep an eye on the alcohol. He recommended and got a Consulting Board of Physicians and Surgeons, which meant he was no longer the only one calling for changes.

During his absence, a separate Penitentiary Hospital building that Sanger had fought for was built and completed. It was so badly constructed, however, it was immediately deemed unfit for occupation. With no one like Sanger in charge to at least try to prevent it, the decision was made to fill

the substandard building with patients anyway. For almost a decade thereafter, the administration argued about how to fix the growing structural
problems.

During Sanger's second term as resident physician he won two
significant battles. A plan was devised that would no longer require people
to be convicted of a crime to be treated there. Sanger also took issue with
the name *Penitentiary Hospital*, which he felt added to the stigma of being
a patient there. Since it would cease functioning as a quasi-penal institution, the name of the hospital was changed to Island Hospital, but the problem of what to do about the dangerously unsound building still loomed.

Early in the morning of February 13, 1858, during a tremendous snow-
storm, a fire started that ended the discussion once and for all. The building
went quickly. Efforts to save the structure had little chance of succeeding,
and strong winds from the northwest rendered them largely useless. To
begin with, the fire hydrants which had been installed throughout the Island didn't work. Rescuers had to run to the river to fill whatever buckets
they could find and pass them along a line of convicts who'd been let out
of their cells by Warden John Fitch. There were no firemen on the line. The
ones who'd shown up at the foot of Sixty-First Street could only stand on
the Manhattan side of the raging and impassable river and watch helplessly
as the flames grew. Sanger lost two years of his prostitution and syphilis
research in the conflagration, but luckily he'd saved an earlier draft of the
book that came out of his work.

The plan to admit people without sentencing them to a crime had
only been devised a few months before, and it had not yet been imple-
mented. So every single patient was locked up inside. Alarms were raised
and keys found, and when they weren't, doors were battered in. Elijah
Simpson, hero to the children of the Colored Orphan Asylum, raced up
a ladder to carry down the hospital matron, who was dressed in only a
nightgown. Soon after, the walls of the Hospital, which had been falling
apart for years and were now held in place by iron straps, burst and fell.
Amazingly, no one perished. One infant died hours later, and while the

smoke and exposure to the elements may have contributed, the baby was already gravely ill.

There was an upside. The destruction of the building presented the commissioners and the Island with a clean slate. The hospital was replaced with a far superior building designed by James Renwick Jr., with modifications by committee, and completed in 1861 (although they started occupying the building the year before).

The new Island Hospital building was now the largest hospital in New York, beating out Bellevue, the original hospital for the poor, in admissions (Bellevue still served the poor, but they focused on accident victims and acute or curable cases). It sat at the southernmost end of the Island, opposite Fifty-First Street in Manhattan, facing its former home, the Penitentiary. The hospital was three and a half stories high, and almost as wide as the Island. When the tides were high and the wind was strong, a sea-salt breeze blew through the wards, sweeping out more objectionable odors.

This would have been the perfect time to enact another of Sanger's repeated proposals, to close down the separate and inferior Almshouse and Workhouse hospitals and treat everyone at one central hospital. But Sanger was unable to consolidate care as he wanted. The Almshouse and Workhouse hospitals remained, as did the top-floor hospital at the Penitentiary, which was now for true convicts alone. Over the coming years more hospitals would arise and fall away as needed, including the Smallpox Hospital, a Fever Hospital, an Epileptic and Paralytic Hospital, a Scarlet Fever Hospital, a Relapsing Fever Hospital, and others. Although patients were often relegated to tents which offered little comfort or protection against inclement weather, for years Blackwell's Island was one of few places that even accepted victims of contagious diseases.

Like all the institutions on Blackwell's Island, administrators sometimes treated available space within the hospitals like a game of musical chairs/beds. The 1880 federal census for the Epileptic and Paralytic Hospital ends with a very intriguing handwritten note. "There is no such institution as an Epileptic & Paralytic Hospital on Blackwell's Island. These people are merely inmates of the Poorhouse placed in certain wards by themselves. I have obtained all the information in regard to them that was possible and reliable. These people are generally of the lowest class, committed by Magistrates for Vagrancy, know or pretend to know nothing in regard to themselves and consequently there is no record of them in this institution, other than that given by me."

Administration of the hospital had already started to go downhill when Sanger resigned for the last time in 1860. The office of the resident physician was inexplicably "dispensed with" and the hospital was once again run by wardens instead of physicians. All the departments: the medical, surgical, gynecological, dermatological, and venereal, were put under the charge of recent graduates who had little experience and no one to turn to for help except the physicians who visited once a week. Workhouse convicts who continued to be employed as nurses and guards pinched whiskey and wine from the apothecary, and went on to run a thriving black market, charging helpless patients for basics like eggs, milk, butter, and blankets. In a few years, wounded and maimed Civil War soldiers began filling up the wards. Veterans whose injuries made them unemployable were sewn up and shuffled off to another institution, their wives and children often to a different one, while the burden on the Department of Public Charities and Correction grew.

The name of the hospital was changed again, in 1866, to Charity Hospital, and a separate medical board was established to oversee all the hospitals on the Island. But the annual reports continued to sound grim. Convalescent patients were put to work: in 1867 they made 504 shrouds. Although the annual report doesn't specifically say they were making shrouds for their fellow patients, there were 505 deaths at Charity Hospital that year.

Among them was a thirty-four-year-old clerk named John Thompson. At four o'clock on Sunday, April 28, orderly Matthew Henderson wrapped a bandage under Thompson's chin and over his head to close his mouth, as was customarily done with the dead. Except Thompson was still breathing, and he made several feeble efforts to turn away from Henderson.

Henderson responded by bracing his back against the wall in order to pull the bandage tighter. Then he kept pressing his fingers against Thompson's eyelids in an attempt to permanently close them. Leave him alone, another patient cried. Let him die in peace. "The man's soul is gone," Henderson replied, "it is only the insides working. I'll do the same to you before long."

Henderson later said he was only joking, and the physician in charge and the warden defended his actions. The charges against him were dropped and he was quietly transferred to Bellevue the following year. Soon after, and without explanation or fanfare, he was removed from his position at Bellevue.

LIFE INSIDE THE relatively new hospital was still bleak the year Rev. French began his mission on Blackwell's Island. Decreases in the patients' diet had been ordered the year before. "I believe that a smaller portion of well-cooked and properly served food would be more beneficial and more acceptable," the chief of staff wrote, "than a larger portion ill-prepared." The following year—French's first—Ann McGeary killed herself by jumping out a window and the next year John Hart cut his own throat. But the downward spiral at Charity began to turn around not long after. Physicians were once again in charge. Heating and ventilation was installed. Planning began for a Lying-In Department for pregnant patients, although some people objected.

The relatively inaccessible Blackwell's Island was not the ideal location for poor women to give birth. Regardless of the time or weather, a woman in labor would have to first travel via horse-driven ambulance to the pier, where she'd board a boat to the Island, before being transferred from the docks to the hospital by carriage or cart. The hospital administrators went ahead with their plans, and in 1874 pregnant women from around the Island and Bellevue were transferred to the newly established department. The administrators didn't stop there. Charity Hospital remained *the* venereal hospital of the city, and the doctors decided that women should not be giving birth so close to people rotting away from syphilis. In 1877

Penitentiary inmates built a separate maternity hospital on the Almshouse grounds, and a new procedure was instituted the following year. Pregnant women were first brought to the Lying-In ward, and when labor began they were moved to one of the two pavilions that made up the maternity hospital.

French never felt as connected to Charity Hospital as he did to other institutions on the Island. The hospital already had an in-house Catholic chaplain, and while it was French's practice to visit and support people of all faiths, the existing hospital chaplain was a dedicated clergyman, too. There was simply less for French to do. But the new maternity pavilions had been built on the Almshouse grounds, where French had his largest and most stable congregation, and where he spent a good deal of his time. Inside those new pavilions he found young mothers who were mere children themselves, many of whom had come to this country alone. They worked as domestic help in family homes and boarding houses, or as maids in hotels, and if they became pregnant they were often thrown out and abandoned. When speaking of the maternity wards, French's hospital reports come alive with fury, as he rebuked the employers who cast the young women aside: "So few masters or mistresses ever imagine that they have any duty to perform to a servant beyond paying their hire."

A messenger came to him one day with an urgent request to minister to a dying mother at one of the pavilions. French found the young woman in a highly agitated state. She confessed to having been a great sinner, but she had repented. "He promises pardon to all who come, does He not?" she asked French anxiously. "I am dying? I know it. . . . So I come to Him for rest. I want to hear Him say to me that He has forgiven me." When she paused for a moment from sheer exhaustion, French began the service that would provide the assurance the terrified woman so desperately craved. She calmed down enough to join him in the Lord's Prayer, but lived only a few moments after French finished the prayer for the dying.

French was livid. These young women were "often more sinned against than sinning," he wrote with sympathy, and they "are in a most pitiable condition, knowing neither where to go, nor what to do." French had to find a way to comfort them. Normally he held services and performed sacraments like Holy Communion as needed, from the hospital chapel at the top of the building. If someone was too sick to be moved or to climb to the stairs he would come to the wards or their bedside.

French came up with a plan to use the baptismal service as a way to show the tiny and forsaken families that they were not all alone in the new world. He looked around and found just the right place to conduct the ceremony, in a pavilion on the river bank, away from the hospital and sickness and death. It took a few trips back and forth to collect all the items he needed to fashion a proper altar. French wanted to be sure to imbue the ceremony with all the dignity and solemnity he felt they deserved. Then he was ready. Everyone was gathered and the infants were anointed from a sterling silver font which he'd placed on a small table covered with "snowy linen vestments." (If the mothers were too ill someone stood in their stead at the ceremony.)

The cobbled-together church couldn't have been more tranquil. In one report French wrote how "last summer, well on towards evening, when the sun was shining brightly in the western window, and a gentle breeze floated in from the river with refreshing coolness," everyone stood around the font, clutching their Bibles, earnestly praying. It was a rare fulfillment of what city planners had envisioned when they first chose Blackwell's Island as the perfect setting for the poor, where all the sick of mind, body, and heart would be restored on this quiet, lush island on the river.

While French was doing what he could to give the new mothers and their babies there a fresh start in life, another group of young women were about to change everything. In 1875, a training school for nurses was launched on Blackwell's Island. The idea of professional, educated nurses was still a very novel development, although nursing schools had already been in operation since 1873 at Bellevue and other hospitals in New England. The two-year program at Blackwell's was open to women between twenty and thirty-five years old who could present certificates affirming their moral character and health. The students lived on the Island and worked as nurses from day one. In between classes in "Poisons and Antidotes," "Midwifery and Children," "Food," "Pulse, Respirations, Temperature, Bandaging, and the Application of Instruments," and "Application of Leeches and Subsequent Treatment," the young women were expected to change bed linens, clean patients, take temperatures, and perform other basic tasks.

After the "the ignorant, unfeeling, and often vicious women" who used to take a washrag to their faces, the new nurses were seen by the patients as the gentlest of angels. Medicine was finally given and temperatures taken, and poultices were applied by women who were tutored and trained. Workhouse women continued to be employed at the Hospital, but once enough nurses had graduated, the Workhouse helpers were relegated to doing laundry and scrubbing the floors, or assisting the nurses who would report any signs of abuse by the Workhouse helpers.

At one of the commencement exercises, a speaker joked that he hoped that after the young women had concluded their service they'd marry the nicest doctor they could find. One of the first graduates, Rose Marvel, married chief of staff Dr. Curtis Estabrook, a doctor so beloved that the people in Canarsie, the working-class neighborhood in Brooklyn where he lived, tried to have Canarsie renamed "Estabrook."

Three members of the first graduating class became briefly notorious as the nurses who cared for Emily Graham, the Lunatic Asylum patient who died in 1879 within forty-eight hours of returning home. Graham's doctor had complained that her remains were filthy and covered in sores. The nurses insisted that she was regularly cleaned and her bed was changed several times a day. Jessie Barber, one of the accused nurses, had even been honored at their graduation for her essay titled "Hygiene."

It would still be some time before Charity lost the reputation as the hospital where people went to die, but during the nurses' second year of classes something else happened that would later spur monumental change. British surgeon Joseph Lister, the father of antiseptic surgery, included Blackwell's

Island on his great American tour of 1876. On October 10, Lister gave a lecture and surgical demonstration at Charity Hospital, in an amphitheater packed with medical students from Bellevue. "Until just now, when I saw you all galloping with such speed from the steamer, I had no idea that I was to address so large a body of students," Lister said, surprised and pleased to see a room full of eager, young doctors of the future.

Lister's method, once it was fully developed, essentially consisted of sterilizing everything. A Blackwell's alumnus later recalled the days when patients were brought in to be operated on "without the slightest attempt at washing the parts in any way. . . . The operator put on an old frock coat which he kept in the operating room for the purpose, and which he buttoned to his chin to protect his clothing from being spattered. It was encrusted with the remains of several years of former operations. . . . Old sponges, unsterilized dressings and constantly infected wards were the rule."

For his demonstration at Charity Hospital, Lister drained—appropriately enough considering the venue—a venereal abscess. Charity Hospital would not be the first to embrace what Lister proposed, but they would be among the hospitals that did it best, devoting a separate room to sterilization, overseen by the operating nurse and kept pristine by the hospital's growing corps of nurses who were now being trained in antiseptic practices.

As time went on, Charity grew into a reasonably good hospital. But despite the new Lying-In Department and Maternity Hospital, pregnant women continued to die at alarming rates. The antiseptic procedures applied so successfully to surgery were not immediately adopted in maternity wards, either in Charity Hospital or in other hospitals across the country. It took a visiting obstetric surgeon, Henry Jacques Garrigues, an immigrant from Denmark, to transfer what they'd learned in surgery to childbirth.

Garrigues began his experiment at Charity Hospital on October 1, 1883, by dividing the wards in the pavilions into "well" and "sick" wards. "Each department had separate doctors, nurses and utensils," leaving Garrigues as the only common element between the two. He then had the doors between the wards locked and sealed. Maternity Hospital doctors and nurses were already forbidden from going to Charity Hospital or the dead house. Garrigues now banned doctors from Charity Hospital. Until then they had often come to the Maternity Hospital "directly from autopsies or septic patients" in order to observe operations. Finally, surgical instruments, doctors, nurses, and wounds were treated using various disinfectants, including those championed by Lister.

In the first nine months in 1883, before Garrigues instituted changes, thirty women died following 345 deliveries. In the twelve months following Garrigues's new practices, "we had 505 deliveries and seven deaths," which commissioners would later describe as "scarcely a single death." Garrigues published his results, which were then adopted nationwide, and he is now considered the father of antiseptic obstetrics. A new, state-of-the-art Maternity Hospital was built on Blackwell's Island in 1888, using Garrigues's plans, replacing the old pavilions on the Almshouse grounds.

Not everything doctors and administrators tried was successful, or even a good idea. In 1876 they tested a new disinfectant for cleaning and deodorizing the wards called Girondin. The primary ingredient of Girondin was copper acetate, which was already known to be poisonous. The product had been condemned by various boards of health in Europe years before, which was reported in the *New York Daily News* in 1871.

In 1879, one doctor injected human milk from a woman in the Lying-In Department into the veins of a twenty-five-year-old woman who had developed abscesses on her ribs due to tuberculosis. She was wasting away from "diarrhea and suppuration" and this action was essentially a Hail Mary pass. The effects from the injection were almost immediate. The patient cried repeatedly about a bad pain in her knee, and one in her chest. But the doctor was more concerned that her pulse rate had gone up, then suddenly plummeted to ten beats a minute. "Take a long breath," he told her.

"I can't," she replied.

Everyone was sure her life was going to end right then and there. The patient rallied, but the doctor announced to all the men gathered in the amphitheater, "She will suffer no harm from the operation, and possibly she may have benefited. However, I think that I have seen enough to convince me that the transfusion of milk should be abandoned. . . . I think we will stick to blood hereafter."

Tuberculosis was frequently the number-one cause of death on the Island, and doctors were always on the lookout for a treatment or cure. In 1886, one doctor injected carbolized iodine (made from combining iodine and carbolic acid) into the lungs of eleven patients, hoping it might act as a disinfectant. The next year another doctor tried the Bergeon Method, which consisted of pumping hydrogen sulfide, a toxic gas that smells like rotten eggs, into the patient's rectum. The theory was the gaseous enema might act as a germicide. "The effect of the use of the gas was rather startling," one doctor commented, after watching one man's stomach quickly swell up "tight as a drum." Neither treatment was effective.

A few years later another doctor conducted a few trials with Aguzon, an ozone preparation taken orally that they also hoped would act as an antiseptic against the disease. Although the doctor reported a good response with patients who were not in advanced stages, no one was cured. If the experiment were to be repeated, he said, they might get better results if the patients were less crowded together and received better food. "A ward in a charity hospital which has held hundreds of consumptives, nearly all of whom have died there, is not the place to hope for the best results." (Over the years scientists have continued to experiment with ozone as a possible treatment, and a number of them have reported positive results.)

Some of the experiments carried out at Charity Hospital had unequivocally horrible outcomes. A letter carrier named William Benson was hypnotized in 1894 instead of receiving anesthesia. Doctors then launched into two hours of brain surgery to remove an abscess. When Benson came to, doctors learned to their horror that he was conscious of everything, every stroke of the saw and the knife, but he could not move, a state which is now referred to as anesthesia awareness.

Two years later another doctor conducted the same experiment, this time on an ex-fireman named Frank Powell. Powell awoke an anguished and broken man. Everyone in the room—assistants, nurses, the doctors watching from the amphitheater—froze as he described the two hours of agony he'd endured as they bored into his skull. "Dr. Bedeau stood speechless by the operating table," a reporter wrote. "Like the accused prisoner before a Court of justice, he unconsciously winced beneath the glaring eyes of the witnesses of his act."

Bedeau recovered quickly. It was all in the "interest of science," he insisted. He invited the observers to "rejoice with me that those of us who have been led into belief in the delusive agency have at least witnessed an exhibition of its treachery and abandon all further idea of its use in surgery." He conveniently left out the fact that his colleague had already provided an equally convincing exhibition years before. (Adam Crabtree, the author of *From Mesmer to Freud: Magnetic Sleep and the Roots of Psychological Healing*, writes, "There are cases of hypnosis being used successfully as an anesthetic during major surgery, and cases where the patient was also conscious during surgery and felt no pain," but not enough is known about these early experiments to speculate about what happened.)

One experiment conducted in 1890, involving a dog named Yip and a fourteen-year-old boy named John Gethins, although certainly well intentioned, seems cruel today. An operation meant to fix the curvature of a bone in Gethins's leg had left an unhealed fracture. In pictures you can see the boy's foot flopping away at the ankle. The case was referred to Dr. Abel M. Phelps, who first attempted to wire the bones together and failed. Doctors in this century would be looking for reasons why the bones of a child were not healing, but back then the next step was amputation. Phelps had told the boy that he'd had some success transplanting bones from a dog. According to Phelps, Gethins started writing to beg him to try this operation on him. Phelps agreed, and Gethins's neighbors in the small town of Horseheads, New York, paid to send him to Charity Hospital for the experimental procedure.

Phelps selected a two-year-old spaniel named Yip, then cut the dog's vocal cords in preparation for the surgery. This was to "relieve the boy from the annoyance of frequent whining," a reporter explained, except it wasn't entirely successful. Witnesses to the operation could hear the dog "moan pitifully." The dog was wrapped in cotton and placed in a sitting position. While an incision was made in the boy's leg, Phelps amputated the paw and around half of one of Yip's legs. Using an aluminum dowel pin and wire, Phelps then attached a section of Yip's bone between the fractured sections of Gethins's leg. Next, the dog was placed beside the boy and the stump of its leg was stitched to the soft parts of the boy's, in the hope that the dog could continue to supply blood to the bone until the boy's blood took over. To prevent movement, Phelps wrapped plaster of Paris around the boy's leg and Yip's entire body, except for his head and tail.

Both the dog and the boy were given an anesthetic during the operation, and Yip was given small doses of morphine afterwards. This was not so much for pain, Phelps explained, as for the anxiety caused by the forced confinement. The dog calmed down after three days, Phelps said, and he and the boy had become friends. If Yip lived, Gethins told a reporter, he was going to take care of him. But the dog turned away when food was offered to him, and he tried, unsuccessfully, to howl.

After eleven days Phelps found "there was an apparent shrinkage of the dog in the dressings." This meant Yip had lost enough weight to give him room to move, which threatened the connection to the boy. The dog was sedated and removed from John. At this point Phelps claimed there was union between the dog bone and the boy's, and both patients were doing fine. At the end of five weeks, however, the decision was made to remove Yip's bone from Gethins's. When the plaster cast was removed Phelps discovered that John's leg was now even shorter that before. He extracted the dog bone, placed the two ends of John's leg "firmly together," and stopped talking to reporters.

There had been a lot of attention in the papers, including angry letters to the editor about the treatment of the dog. One writer pointed out that

Phelps had performed unnecessary and barbaric experiments on dogs before, and had been censured by his colleagues. In a previous experiment to learn about bone rigidity, four dogs were ultimately killed only to confirm what Phelps himself conceded was already known about what he was studying. Not only were the experiments therefore unnecessary, they were conducted without anesthesia. About one dog, Phelps wrote that he "did very well for a few weeks. . . . But at the end of the fifth week he refused to eat and began to emaciate. A week later . . . he was killed. An excoriation, due to pressure, was found below the knee upon removing the dressing. This accounted for the loss of appetite, as much pain must have been induced." This meant Phelps knew that one likely cause of Yip's loss of appetite was pain.

The following March Phelps published his own paper about the Gethins experiment, reporting what was already known, that the operation had failed. Phelps insisted that Yip did not suffer except for the "uneasiness" of confinement, and added that he'd successfully reconnected the dog's vocal cords, restoring Yip's ability to bark and howl.

One of Phelps' goals with the Gethins operation was to demonstrate that the soft parts of an animal could be transplanted to a man. His list of possible cases for which this technique might be applied, like the "scalps ripped from the heads of factory girls by machinery," addresses distinctly nineteenth-century hazards, but also shows some measure of compassion. Over a century later, Dr. Leonard F. Peltier would write, "Although there are many anecdotes of allografts [grafts involving skin, bone, ligaments, etc.] Dr. Phelps's account is unique because it also incorporates the idea of using a vascularized graft." Vascularized bone grafts are used today to repair exactly the problem Gethins presented.

Six months after the operation John Gethins met with a reporter in the local barber shop of Joe Smith, the man responsible for raising the money to send him to New York. The boy's face was pale and he looked like he hadn't slept. Gethins claimed that Phelps had told him when it was all over "he was going to have me sent to school and educated and afterwards would have me study medicine and become a doctor." The poor son of a tenant farmer had briefly nurtured a dream that he would have his leg back, and a whole new elevated life. But when it was clear that the operation had failed, Phelps sent him back to Horseheads instead, telling him that his "leg may yet come out all right." Gethins was left with a future more bleak than before. He still had his leg, but it was even shorter now, which left him incapable of manual labor, his likely only option for making a living. The article ends without answers or assurance for a frightened boy who didn't know what was going to "become of him."

Ten years later Gethins was working at St. John's Catholic Protectory, an orphanage in Erie, New York, where he started out as a guard and ended up a teacher. Somehow he managed to put together the education his father couldn't afford to give him, and that Phelps had allegedly retreated from his promise to provide. Abel M. Phelps died following abdominal surgery in 1902. He was fifty-one. Neither Phelps, any reporters, or Gethins, ever recorded what became of Yip.

In 1892, by order of the Commissioners of the Department of Public Charities and Correction, Charity Hospital was renamed yet again. It became City Hospital. Rev. French was by this time concentrating his missionary efforts on the Lunatic Asylum and the Almshouse. City Hospital was seen to by a succession of replacement priests, none of whom seemed to particularly care for the work. French's first successor, Rev. Gustav W. Mayer, admitted to wearying of the responsibilities. "The giving out of sympathy is very exhaustive, and sometimes when, after a hard day's work, I begin another day's work, I don't feel one bit like beginning it. I shrink from it, and would give almost anything if only my conscience suffered me to shirk the work. I am sorry this is so, *but it is so*, and I am bound to make a public confession of it right here." Rev. Braddin Hamilton, who followed Mayer, wrote that "the work in the crowded wards is anything but pleasant, where we have to inhale so much of the close atmosphere." Apparently the efforts to eradicate the smells were not entirely successful.

Part of the problem French's colleagues were experiencing was that the general lack of "visible, definite results" led to burnout and despair. Like French, the priests longed to see the fruits of their labors. "I am not certain of my ministry having affected permanently the life and conduct of a single soul found amidst the tides of humanity that have surged through these wards," the Rev. Hugh Maguire, another relief priest, confided. What were they dragging themselves to work for?

Maguire actually preferred the Penitentiary to City Hospital. "There are not the same sad and awful sights to behold, not the same piercing and horrible cries to be heard." Even though City Hospital had come a long way, it was still a hospital, and this was still the nineteenth century. A lot of the people Maguire visited died. The first person buried in the new potter's field on Hart Island came from Charity Hospital (Louisa Van Slyke, who died of tuberculosis on April 10, 1869). After the Almshouse, Charity Hospital was the chief source of bodies bound for the potter's field from Blackwell's Island.

But at the Penitentiary, Maguire said, "the prisoners are healthy, active and vigorous. A larger proportion would seem to be more easily reached by the Gospel and permanently reformed, than is found among the moral waifs and wrecks flooding the Hospital." The Penitentiary was also one of the more democratic institutions on the Island. You didn't have to be poor to stay there, although many—almost certainly most—prisoners were.

One of the prisoners Rev. French would have come across on his daily rounds at the Penitentiary was the very priest he'd replaced when he arrived at Blackwell's in 1872, the Rev. Edward Cowley. While other priests recoiled from the work at the Hospital, Cowley threw himself and his family right into the thick of it by moving onto the grounds with his wife in July of 1864, towards the end of the Civil War. He did this in order to be more immediately available to the soldiers who'd started arriving, and to the sick and dying in general. They lived there until Cowley left to pursue the private charitable work which would eventually land him in the Penitentiary. The charge: cruelty to children.

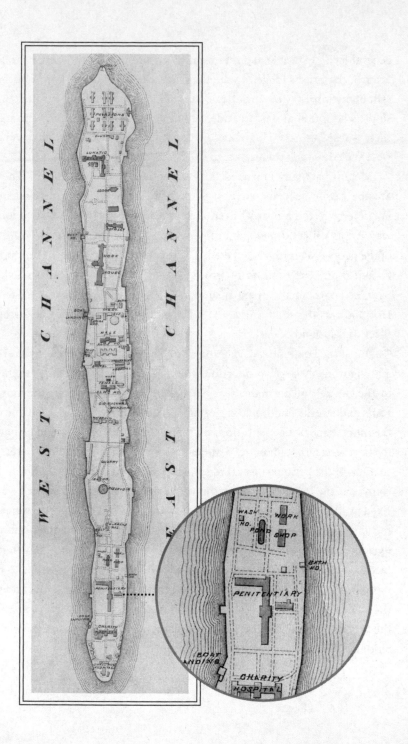

THE PENITENTIARY

COMPLETED IN 1832, FOR PEOPLE CONVICTED
OF MORE SERIOUS CRIMES, AND WITH SENTENCES
GENERALLY FROM THREE TO SIX MONTHS TO
TWO YEARS, ALTHOUGH SOMETIMES MORE

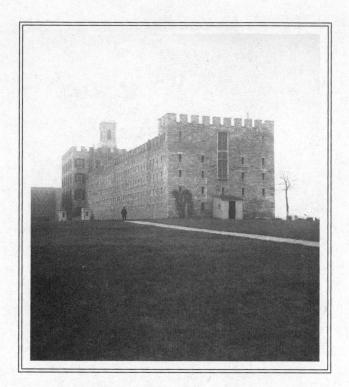

ADELAIDE IRVING

Sentenced to the Penitentiary December 6, 1862

THE BLACKWELL'S ISLAND Penitentiary, where many of the most inveterate criminals of New York City were sent, offered Rev. French his best shot at something he expressed a longing for in almost every report: to see with his own eyes that he'd actually helped someone turn their life around. Every year, thousands of people he worked with on the Island "passed out of sight," he wrote, without ever granting him the satisfaction of knowing that the seeds he had sown had grown. The lunatics often sank further, and hospital patients died. Workhouse inmates came and went too quickly for French to even make an impression. But prisoners in the Penitentiary were comparatively healthy, and had longer sentences.

In his 1879–1880 annual report, French related a story of achieving what he yearned for most. That year, a former inmate of the Island spotted French in the streets of Manhattan. The man jumped down from the wagon he was riding in and grabbed French's hand. "I have watched often to see you," the man cried. "Don't you know me? I was over there," he said, pointing towards the East River. One day, following a chapel service, French had found this man in tears, and he had taken his hand to give him words of encouragement. Now he grasped the hand of a thriving and utterly altered man. French was as elated as his former congregant. I'm so glad "to see you prospering," French said. "Yes, I am prospering," the man answered, still holding his former priest's hand, each thrilled to see the other again under such different circumstances. "What you said to me put me on the right track. I have been living, and mean to live an honest life, and I wanted to tell you so."

French needed that win. Charles Loring Brace, who ministered to the sick on Blackwell's Island (and who would go on to found the Children's Aid Society) once wrote his sister, "You can have no idea, Emma, what an immense vat of misery and crime and filth much of this great city is!" With up to nearly a quarter of its average daily population of seven thousand dying yearly, some through murder, suicide, or neglect, small victories like this one held French up as he watched so many others sink, regardless of everything he did to try to save them.

IN THE SUMMER of 1879, the same year that French ran into the former Penitentiary inmate, a reporter in search of a story climbed the steep hill to the old burying ground at Sing Sing, a notoriously brutal state prison along the Hudson River, and said to be the source of the phrase *sent up the river*. On the southern end of the cemetery was a long-neglected grave covered in pink wildflowers and marked with two white sticks that had become entangled with vines. He pulled the foliage aside. A single hand-painted name could still be read on the crude marker: *Addie*. Addie, he would explain to his readers, was "remembered by New York detectives as one of the worst female thieves that ever infested the metropolis." She'd been sentenced under the name Rebecca A. Fitch, but she also frequently used the alias Adelaide Irving, and the nickname Addie. Whoever painted her name on her grave marker, the reporter theorized, must have chosen Addie as the "safest guess and most cautious inscription."

In all the times that she had been admitted and discharged from Sing Sing, Addie had never provided a name or address for her next of kin. When she died in 1870, two years before her sentence was up, they placed her in a convict-built coffin and buried her on a bluff to the northeast of the prison, near a single tree, a few shrubs, and a profusion of weeds, which, by the time the reporter visited, had already covered over most of the forgotten graves there.

It was such a desolate patch of land that the reporter was moved to ask, What was it like, to sicken and die in such a place? Perhaps to ease his mind, a doctor told him that when convicts are near death they are indifferent. But he added, "The time when they have the horrors is when they are afraid they are going to be sick enough to die," at which point they are like anyone else—terrified. We'll never know Addie's state of mind as she lay dying, but sometime before, she wrote to Mrs. Elizabeth Buchanan, a prison visitor who had befriended her, "Oh God! I wish I was a child again, innocent & free from guilt."

Addie, whose real name was, in fact, Adelaide Irving, was only twenty-three years old when she died. She was so far from being the worst female thief in New York that the flagrant exaggeration is more likely due to a desperate need to sell newspapers, or vanity, than anything else. She'd made a couple of relatively small mistakes when she was young, and due to the obliviousness of youth and the assumption that life would go on forever, she never noticed that the tendrils of justice had already wrapped themselves around her future, and the slow, inexorable descent into the earth on this lonely precipice had begun.

On June 7, 1862, her fifteenth birthday, Addie was riding the nineteenth-century version of public transportation—a horse-drawn stagecoach called an omnibus—when she pulled the strap to request her stop and slipped out the door. In what was likely an automatic gesture in those relatively lawless times, the woman sitting near her patted her pocket and discovered her wallet was missing. She ran off after Addie. A few months later, Addie was brought before Recorder John T. Hoffman in the Court of General Sessions to explain why the woman's wallet was found in her possession (a recorder was an elected judicial official, empowered as a judge in the Court of General Sessions).

Over 150 years later, her answer, that she'd found the wallet, still doesn't ring true. The contents were valued at $6.11, and Addie was declared guilty of petit larceny, a crime that normally would have landed her for a brief time in the Workhouse or the Penitentiary. But she was just a child. And an attractive one. A reporter who covered the courts described her as a "very pretty, fat [cheeked] girl." Addie was also a well-brought-up young woman, although she'd always been, she would admit, quite willful. She'd come to New York the year before and was so enthralled by the city she refused to return home. She was taken in by her uncle, who found her a job as a sales girl.

Hoffman decided to give Addie a break and suspended her sentence. Don't do it again, he instructed Addie as he let her go.

A month and a half later Addie was back in court on similar charges. This time they skipped the trial and, based on her prior conviction, Hoffman sent her to the Penitentiary for two years. It was an outrageous sentence. It was severe even for the more hardened and habitual criminals typically sentenced to the Penitentiary, never mind a fifteen-year-old girl who was being imprisoned for the first time, for a minor offense. Although long sentences for equivalent crimes were not unheard of, most people who were sentenced to the Penitentiary for petit larceny were given sentences of six months or less. Hoffman's sentencing history was no different. In all the other reported cases of petit larceny he'd sat on that year, he never sentenced anyone to more than six months. Why throw the book at Addie? Young pickpockets were notoriously hard to catch—maybe Hoffman wanted to make an example of the one they'd managed to arrest. Twice. Addie also seems to have been sentenced at the beginning of a wave of zero tolerance for girls. The next year no less than forty-two girls under fifteen were sent to the Penitentiary. Or it could be that Hoffman simply felt he'd been played by the pretty young thing, and the punitive sentence soothed his damaged ego. (Hoffman would go on to become mayor, then governor of New York, but his political career would be destroyed by his association with Boss Tweed.)

By the time Addie got to the Penitentiary, it was far from the place Rev. Stanford had predicted at the cornerstone ceremony would guide convicts in "the paths of virtue." The Penitentiary was now famous as a training ground for criminals. Recorder Hoffman had to have known reform was the last thing that would take place during Addie's time there. He knew the kinds of people he and his fellow judges were sending there every day. He was also well aware of who worked there.

For one brief moment it looked like Addie just might avoid that grave-yard on the hill. Fifteen men had "eloped" (escaped) from the Penitentiary during her first year there, and one girl: Addie. For Addie it was also an elopement as we understand the word today. Like many convicts before her, Addie had been shuffled around on the Island. While serving part of her sentence in the Workhouse, she met and fell in love with Isaac Fitch, the son of the warden, John Fitch. They were both sixteen years old, but young Isaac was kind and respectful to Addie, and protective. He told her the Island was no place for her and helped her to escape.

Three weeks later, on November 3, 1863, they were married at the most fashionable church in New York City, Trinity Church. Later, few would believe that the marriage had actually taken place. Everyone just assumed that the name Fitch was an alias. But the records are still there, in the Trinity Church archives. The young couple did not get much time together. Within a few weeks, Addie was recaptured and sent back to the Island to finish her sentence, and Isaac was packed off to serve as a private in the Union Army.

Sometime later, Joseph Keen, the Penitentiary warden, came to Addie's cell, accompanied by an officer. "Here is a gentleman your mother sent to see you." Keen turned to the man and said, "she is not naturally wayward, only a lover of mischief." The officer asked if he could meet with Addie alone and Keen brought them to the reception room. When Keen left, the officer bolted the door and turned to Addie. "You know what I am here for," he said, and tried to kiss her. Addie would later say that he told her if she "submitted to him he would give me a ladies [sic] life and I need never steal again, he would have me pardoned and gratify my least wish." Addie refused and served out her sentence.

She was out for a mere eight months before she was sentenced again, in 1865. This time she'd stolen clothes and a pair of boots valued at $50, a more substantial amount, and the charge was grand larceny. The *New York Herald* published a story claiming that Addie's mother had taught her how to steal, and that the eye infection she was suffering from during her trial was the result of syphilis (which they referred to genteelly as "her imprudent conduct"). Adelaide wrote a letter to the paper. She was the youngest of six girls, and all her sisters had married well. She considered her mother's parenting and asked, if she had "trained me in the art of thieving, why were not the rest of her children trained so?" As far as the charges about her conduct, she renounced them completely and challenged her accusers to provide evidence of her licentiousness.

Addie telegraphed Isaac in Washington, who rushed back and once again tried to rescue her. He met with Addie's victim and begged her to drop the charges. The woman refused. Addie pled guilty and threw herself at the mercy of the court. But the court was represented by the previously merciless Recorder Hoffman. This time he upped the ante and sentenced Addie to three years in the prison for the most hardened criminals of all, Sing Sing. It was, again, an unusually harsh sentence. According to the Women's Prison Association, 5,934 women were sent from New York City to Blackwell's Island in 1866 (they didn't supply numbers for 1865), while only twenty-six women were sent to Sing Sing. Addie was now eighteen years old.

When she was released three years later in 1868, she'd already spent five years of her life in prison. She was free for nine months before she was arrested for the last time. The clothing and jewelry she'd stolen was valued at $69, and bail was set at $2,500.

By 1868, Addie was alone. She'd become estranged from her family. Although there appear to be no records of a divorce or an annulment, while Addie was serving her sentence in Sing Sing, Isaac had wed a sixteen-year-old girl named Catherine. (Isaac and Catherine had three sons before Isaac died in 1887, when he was forty.) Addie's only friends were her fellow criminals, and they couldn't come up with $2,500. Her counsel didn't even try to mount a real defense. He only argued that her crime was petit larceny, not grand larceny. The judge (not Hoffman) sentenced her to another three years in Sing Sing. Two weeks after arriving to serve her second and final prison sentence, Addie turned twenty-two. She'd be dead within a year.

"I was a good, virtuous girl when I first saw the cell door closed on me, on the Island," she wrote to the *New York Herald*, referring to Blackwell's Island, before her first sentence at Sing Sing. And "I may thank the Island for all my trouble." From the moment she entered the Penitentiary, Addie insisted, "Sing Sing was my doom." Blackwell's was famous as a stepping stone to greater crimes, and still more barbaric prisons, and most reformers would agree with Addie that inmates were dragged under rather than rehabilitated there. However Addie was still feeling hopeful the day she penned that letter. "But I am not gone yet," she wrote about Sing Sing, "and maybe won't go." She went.

Addie was still as naive as she'd been at fifteen. From her cell in Sing Sing she wrote blissfully to Mrs. Buchanan about the day of Salvation, and "won't it be beautiful when we shall meet our Savior. . . . I won't be a convict then, Mrs. B." It was the tone of someone who had no idea how quickly she would be put underground to wait.

Nothing remains of the cemetery where she was buried, although some of the bodies were moved in the 1940s. Not Addie's. The two white sticks which marked her grave in 1870s were almost certainly long gone, and no one knew she was down there.

TWO YEARS AFTER Addie died, Rev. French stepped inside the place where the once pretty and cheeky young woman had begun her steady slide to oblivion. French agreed with reformers, and wrote that "if any man, or set of men should try to find the best possible plan to educate criminals, they could not find one more effectual to that end than the one in existence in this Institution." Today, criminal justice authorities call prisons "graduate school for crime."

It's hard to even imagine a fifteen year old inside such a place. The anarchist Johann Most, who was sentenced to Blackwell's Island twice, would call it "the true Siberia of America." Addie would have been assigned with another woman to a cell that, at six feet nine inches high, three and a half feet wide, and seven feet deep, couldn't be said to be humanely big enough for one. They called it a cell, "but 'trench' would be a more explicit term," Most wrote. "These prison lodgings are simply caves in the granite," without light, air, or heat. There were no windows, and along each passage outside there was only one gaslight every fifty feet, and a single stove for warmth. The cells were without furniture except for two strips of canvas that served as their beds, and these came with blankets that would not be washed during their entire stay. The only other items in their cells were a tin cup for drinking and a chamber pot. Every morning they were led to the river on what Johann Most called "the parade of excrement buckets," where the contents were dumped and the pails rinsed (in violation of an existing health ordinance).

The hall where they took their meals was similarly lightless and gloomy. "Owing to the darkness of the prison," a *New York Times* reporter wrote in 1875, "a huge reflector lamp, facing the long row of tables, is lighted at meal times." An evening school was established that year, offering classes in reading, writing, and arithmetic, but two years later the warden wrote, "We have occasionally been obliged to omit holding the school on account of the poor quality and inadequate supply of gas furnished to this Institution. As soon as this is remedied, and a better supply is furnished, the school can be regularly held."

The stone and iron Penitentiary was the most imposing structure on the Island. Looking towards the opposite shore of Manhattan, it stretched from a little below Fifty-Fifth Street to just below Fifty-Seventh. Like the Lunatic Asylum, the crenelated pattern along the rooftops of the Penitentiary made it look like a castle, in this case a long drawn-out castle roughly in the shape of a cross. The Penitentiary was the first institution built on the Island, and the first to suffer from overcrowding.

There was a reason they didn't anticipate the criminal housing shortage. Their initial vision was "to season justice with mercy." But mercy had a price. Except for the crimes of treason, murder, and arson, imprisonment for the penitent had replaced capital punishment in New York City. By the time they were done building, the Penitentiary, which was originally supposed to contain 240 cells, grew to 496 cells. That should have been sufficient for as far into the future as they could imagine, except criminals that previously would have been either killed or banished had to go somewhere. It wasn't long before cells meant for one man were housing two, and another 240 cells added later would not eliminate the need for doubling up.

The city planners also did not foresee the explosion in the number of females being sent to prison. New categories of crimes, defined by the very strict codes of behavior for women, meant that "disorderly conduct" could mean just about anything society currently disapproved of, like lesbianism. A woman could be sent away for five years for giving a man a blow job, while the recipient was sent on his merry way.

By 1873 the average daily population in the Penitentiary had climbed to 865, and from there it would keep climbing.

The proximity of the city was as tortuous for the Penitentiary convicts as it was for the other inmates of Blackwell's Island. When recommending they build a wall to limit the number of escapees, the warden added that "the sound and sight of music and dancing on the New-York shore has a tendency to make the prisoners very discontented." A reduced sightline to paradise might alleviate their torment, and the compulsion to bolt.

Something needed to be done because convicted criminals were demonstrably more resourceful than lunatics at getting off the Island. They'd enlist their friends to row over under the cover of darkness, while bribing a keeper to either help them or look the other way. Sometimes they'd get the coxswain drunk and then commandeer the Department of Public Charities and Correction rowboat and row back to Manhattan themselves.

Most of the escapes were from the Workhouse, where many inmates were able to move about the Island relatively freely, making it that much

simpler to make their getaway. In 1866, 546 inmates successfully fled the
Workhouse. The worst year for the Penitentiary was 1867, when they had
seventy-nine escapes. But new wardens in both the Workhouse and the
Penitentiary managed to bring the numbers down sharply in the late 1870s,
and by the 1880s escapes were down to single digits in both institutions.

Some believed there were fewer escapes from the Penitentiary because
the Penitentiary was not such a bad place to be. In 1852, Joseph Keen wrote
that "were it really a 'terror to evil doers,' or a school of reform—there
should be a constant decrease in the number of its inmates. . . . It would
not be the convenient, occasional resort of the scum of our city . . . in their
hours of want and weariness. Yet such is its character." In *A Pickpocket's
Tale: The Underworld of Nineteenth-Century New York*, Timothy J. Gilfoyle
writes that inmates and reformers "alike sarcastically referred to the Blackwell's Island Penitentiary as the 'Old Homestead.'"

That may have been the experience for some, but all things weren't
equal inside, and life there changed for everyone under the rather severe
and heartless Louis D. Pilsbury, who took over as warden in 1886. Pilsbury
routinely threw people in a dark cell, or "cooler" (the names for solitary),
where they'd open the doors daily, according to Johann Most biographer
Frederic Trautmann, to check if the inmate was alive, "loony," or dead.

People were sentenced to the Penitentiary from either the Court of
General Sessions or the Court of Special Sessions. Although many of the
sentences were for six months and under, this was New York City's penal
institution for mid-range sentences, which could span anywhere from one
to ten years. People with sentences over ten years went to Sing Sing and
Auburn, although there are exceptions. Women with longer sentences, including life, for arson or murder, could be sent to Blackwell's.

Once sentenced, prisoners were piled into a carriage called the Black
Maria, which took them from the Tombs to the dock at Twenty-Sixth
Street, where they boarded a steamer. The pier at Twenty-Sixth Street
had evolved into a grim and dangerous place, and for a long time visitors
and city employees called for a police guard to chase away criminals who

lurked about, looking for recruits. Later, the walk to the pier would be referred to as "Misery Lane."

The Penitentiary admission process wasn't much different than it was for every other institution on the Island. Convicts were brought into a large reception room on the ground floor, where the hall keeper sat at a desk on a raised platform. Their name, place of birth (from the later half of the 1860s on, native born Americans outnumbered the Irish in the Penitentiary), age, religion, and occupation were noted along with their crime and sentence. If they'd been there before, including under different names, that would be noted as well, along with their height, weight, and any distinguishing marks, scars or tattoos.

In the same large room were several baths and barber chairs. After they were stripped, cleaned, trimmed, and shaven, the men were given a suit of prison stripes, reducing them to the look of what Charles Dickens called "faded tigers." The women went through a similar intake elsewhere, which in their case ended with them donning striped dresses which somehow managed to look less prison-like.

Female prisoners with infants were allowed to bring them along, and part of the Penitentiary Hospital was partitioned off as a lying-in room for women who were expecting. Children either brought to or born in the prison would remain there until they were weaned, when they were transferred to Randalls Island, or to family or friends.

Every day the men and women were awoken before dawn. They were given two to five minutes at a shared tank to wash themselves, and one towel was distributed to every fifty inmates. Breakfast consisted of bread and weak coffee. Then it was off to work. The women kept the prison clean, and did most of the sewing and the laundry. The men were put in gangs and sent off to the blacksmith workshop or the boathouse, or out to repair or construct buildings, sea walls, and roads. During the day, guard boats with two prisoners to row and a coxswain armed with a carbine and a revolver circled the Island.

In the evening, three night watchmen walked along the tiers armed with a gun and a lantern. If there were any problems, like a discrepancy in the evening prisoner count, a telegraph connected to the warden's residence (a short distance away), the office of the commissioners of the Department of Public Charities and Correction, police headquarters at Mulberry Street, and the Nineteenth Precinct at Fifty-Ninth Street, could summon help.

John Fitch, whose son married Adelaide Irving, was the warden of the Penitentiary when Rev. French arrived. French never mentioned Fitch in his annual reports, which was unusual. French usually managed a kind word for those in charge. It could be that the two men did not hit it off; others had a problem with Fitch. Dr. William Sanger and Warden Fitch famously did not get along. Fitch once tried to hold Sanger responsible for the escape of seven prisoners and his claim was reported in the newspapers. "There was palpable lack of harmony between the Warden and Dr. Sanger," the *New York Times* wrote.

The Penitentiary was suffering from a lot of bad press in French's first years, and at the end of 1874 a grand jury conducted an investigation. Among other issues they were looking into, there had been claims that Boss Tweed, who'd been convicted of multiple counts of fraud and sent to the Penitentiary the year after French arrived, was receiving preferential treatment. He was in a room and not a cell, and he had a relatively cushy assignment as an orderly in the Penitentiary Hospital. The commissioners would use Tweed's large size—he was said to weigh over 300 pounds—and the state of his health to defend his quarters and the job he was given, and while no charges were brought against them, all three commissioners were soon replaced.

John M. Fox replaced Fitch as the warden at the beginning of 1875. He began his tenure convinced that he could accomplish some good there, so it's no surprise that French and Fox got along. The Penitentiary was without a library when French first arrived and Fox supported his efforts to create one, seeing it as a measure of reform.

Under Fox's management, a new blacksmith workshop was constructed, and the roof, which leaked during every storm, was repaired. Fox also recommended constructing additional accommodations for the women. "We have plenty of stone on the island, and a wing could easily be built," he wrote. Fox was the one who'd established the evening school at the Penitentiary. He also did what he could to make sure that the downward trajectory of a young person like Addie Fitch never happened again.

According to Fox, the current statute decreed that no one under sixteen could be incarcerated in the Penitentiary. Fox checked the admission books. Six prisoners under sixteen were found, including one girl, Jennie Lewis. Jennie's lawyer had asked that she be sent to the House of Refuge, but Judge Sutherland insisted on sending her to the Penitentiary. Part of the problem, Fox maintained, was that the magistrates made no effort to verify the ages of the people they sentenced; they merely guessed, while many adolescents contributed to the problem by lying about their ages. Young people actually preferred the Penitentiary. At the House of Refuge they could be held indefinitely. At least in the Penitentiary their sentences had a fixed end date. Fox also did what he could to separate the young offenders from the old, so that there would be "no opportunity to be poisoned by coming in contact with the hardened criminal."

French always generously credited Fox for helping him in his mission. "The present warden, Mr. Fox, does all in his limited sphere for the welfare of the prison, and welcomes all efforts to do the inmates good."

The operative word there is "limited." French would sadly relate that "for a short time a night school was carried on by prison teachers, but it did not succeed." The "young and old offenders," whom Fox had tried to separate, were now able to interact freely and "corrupt each other without restraint."

Keeping children out of prison proved to be an insurmountable challenge. In the 1868 book *The Secrets of the Great City: A Work Descriptive of the Virtues and the Vices, the Mysteries, Miseries and Crimes of New York City*, James D. McCabe Jr. wrote, "The Commissioners of Public Charities and Correction, in their last report, made the startling announcement that there are no less than thirty-nine thousand children in the City of New

York, growing up in ignorance and idleness." The commissioners were referring both to orphans on the street and to children of poor and profligate parents. Without intervention, many were doomed. "At ten the boys are thieves, at fifteen the girls are all prostitutes." Despite Fox's efforts, judges persisted in sending young people to the Penitentiary. While a new 1877 law provided for the removal of children under fourteen, not sixteen, 141 vulnerable prisoners from fourteen to seventeen years old remained, and more kept coming every year.

In 1879, the year French ran into the thriving ex-con, an inmate named Christie Snyder was murdered by keeper (aka prison guard) Michael Adams. In a June 10, 1879, article the *New York Herald* accused Warden Fox of covering up the keeper's involvement in the death. Later that year they would also charge him with lax management that allowed prisoners to escape. The truth was there were only ten escapes that year, and Fox was responsible for bringing the numbers down. The keepers who were found to have facilitated escapes had not been hired by him, but by the commissioners, and like every other employee on the Island, they could only be fired by them.

French's optimism about the Penitentiary continued to plummet, and by the next annual report he doesn't mention it at all.

WILLIAM H. RAMSCAR

The Old Gentlemen's Unsectarian Home
Sentenced to the Penitentiary December 23, 1889

———————◆———————

POLICE OFFICER DANIEL Fitzpatrick was walking his beat at 3 a.m. on the morning of March 15, 1882, when he spotted a prowler on the grounds of the Old Gentlemen's Unsectarian Home, a private institution occupying a mansion on the top of a hill at the corner of 165th Street and Mott Avenue in the south Bronx. It was a bucolic spot at the time. Although the institution was listed as a "House of Rest for Consumptives and Home for Incurables," they took in anyone who was willing to pay, and they'd started taking in healthy children the previous summer. The charges were $4 a month per child; the children of widows were admitted at a cut rate of $2 a month. It was such a small amount, even for the time, that poor, working parents must have congratulated themselves on being able to send their children to what was thought of as the country so cheaply.

Fitzpatrick climbed through a basement window and into the laundry in order to investigate what he thought was a possible burglary. Inside he found two workers, Susan Hall and Ellen McMasters, and three little girls sleeping. One of the girls started screaming, and while Fitzpatrick attempted to calm her, Ellen McMasters ran upstairs to wake William H. Ramscar, the secretary and superintendent of the home. Instead of being grateful for the officer's actions, Ramscar, a short, stout, forty-nine-year-old native of England, marched down to police headquarters the next day to complain that Officer Fitzpatrick had trespassed on his property.

A reporter from the *Sun*, William R. Benjamin, got wind of the alleged prowler and the subsequent complaint, and visited the home the next afternoon. He would later say that "when I entered the dining-room there was the most terrible stench, it was simply unendurable. . . . I could not breathe in the dining-room." Benjamin talked to the girls who were sleeping in the laundry when the policeman had entered. He noticed that all the children had sore throats and seemed sick, but as far as he was concerned there was no story here.

Seven children had died so far that year inside those walls. In the remaining two weeks of March, three more children would die.

Later on the day Benjamin had visited, one of the women Officer Fitzpatrick had encountered in the laundry room that night, Susan Hall, quit. She'd been hired as a laundress but was instead put to work in the nursery. It was so miserable working among all the dying children she'd only lasted two months. The other woman, Ellen McMasters, had just started working there. She'd been hired as a cook, but on her first day, instead of sending her to the kitchen, they told her to wash and lay out a child who had recently died. Ellen McMasters was made of stronger stuff. She took care of the dead child and was promoted to nurse later in May.

Samuel Warburton, who had two daughters in the home, aged six and eight years old, came to the home on March 11 to take his youngest to the dentist. He was so alarmed by her condition he sent his son back for his other daughter. Tell Ramscar that if he gives you any trouble, he instructed his son, I'm going to the newspapers. The child came home infested with vermin, but alive.

The next month a new boarder, Emma McGee, made a deal with Ramscar to work in the nursery in exchange for her room and board. On her second day a six-month-old infant named Charles Shutz died of ulcerative stomatitis, aka trench mouth. This is not usually a fatal disease, but left untreated, as it most surely was in this case, it can lead to death. The baby may also have stopped eating due to the pain, and that could have been a contributing cause. His bottom was so raw and sore that when Mrs. Ramscar asked Emma to wash the little one and prepare him for burial she couldn't bring herself to do it. The "sight of the child was too much for me," she would later testify. So Charles was left to lie there. "Nobody bothered," she said.

Unlike the other women, Emma didn't hesitate to bring her concerns about the children's care to the attention of Ramscar and his wife, Margaret. The babies were being fed milk that was so curdled, she told them, that "they could not draw the milk through the tubes . . . the tube was so completely stopped." She also pointed out that the milk bottles were being washed in the same basin they used to clean the children. According to Emma, the Ramscars weren't interested. "I never saw Mr. or Mrs. Ramscar pay any attention whatever to the children, if they were very sick, he would say 'that little baby won't live just let it lie there.'" The Ramscars not only ignored Emma's protests, they told her she had to find some place else to live because she was making too much of a disturbance. The death toll, meanwhile, had climbed to eleven.

Later that same month, on the evening of April 18, a little boy named John Hamill was found wandering aimlessly a little over a half mile away from the Unsectarian Home. A beat cop was summoned and John was taken to police headquarters and later to the Lost Children's Department. In the police report, John was described as so "terribly diseased" his feet were literally rotting away, and he could barely stand. The boy told them his father's name was Hugh, and that his mother was dead, but beyond that, nothing more could be learned from him. The police decided to take him to the New York Society for the Prevention of Cruelty to Children (NYSPCC). The Society had more experience with children. Perhaps they could find out where he came from.

The New York Society for the Prevention of Cruelty to Children was a relatively new organization. It had formed in 1874 after Henry Bergh, the founder of the American Society for the Prevention of Cruelty to Animals, and Elbridge T. Gerry, counsel for the ASPCA, started looking into the case of an abused toddler named Mary Ellen. Mary Ellen's widowed mother had been paying another woman, Mary Score, to board and care for her. When Mary Ellen's mother lost her job and stopped making payments, Score took the child to the office of the Superintendent of Outdoor Poor, who sent her on to Blackwell's Island.

Mary Ellen was living in the Almshouse, which in all probability would have resulted in the death of the eighteen-month-old, when a couple looking for a child to indenture selected her and took her home. An indenture is a contract entered into with, in this case, the Department of Public Charities and Correction. A child was bound out as a servant or an apprentice, and in return the child had to be fed, cared for, educated, and taught a skill. At the end of the indenture the child was sent off with a new suit of clothes and a Bible.

There are indications on Mary Ellen's indenture contract, however, that from the point of view of the family removing her, this was an adoption and not an indenture. All the terms referring to indenture were crossed out and filled in with terms describing an adoption. For instance, *Apprentice* was crossed out and replaced with *Child*. *Master* was replaced with *Parent*. It was later claimed that the man adopting Mary Ellen was her biological father. Her abuse began when the man died and she fell under the care of his wife and her new husband.

A missionary who had been investigating the charges of cruelty towards Mary Ellen soon discovered that you could do almost anything you wanted to a child at the time, short of murder or sexual relations. The existing laws did little to deter you. The missionary turned to Bergh for help. This ultimately led to a trial, the founding of the NYSPCC, and ongoing advocacy for better laws and protections for children. In 1876, a year after the NYSPCC incorporated, two men and seven women were the first to be sent to the Penitentiary for cruelty to children.

Edward F. Jenkins, the superintendent of the NYSPCC, accepted John Hamill from the police, and after learning that the boy had come from the Old Gentlemen's Unsectarian Home, he sent him upstairs to his wife to be cleaned up. When Mrs. Jenkins called down in alarm, Jenkins ran up and discovered just how bad the boy's condition was. His body was "one mass of sores and scabs under which the vermin were working," and his left leg was so putrefied and decayed it "was almost rotted off." Jenkins immediately sent John to Bellevue and from there he was put on a steamer to the children's hospital on Randalls Island.

A few days earlier, two-month-old Minnie Smith became the twelfth child to die at the Unsectarian Home. While Jenkins and his wife were discovering just how bad John Hamill's condition was, Adele Fogrolle brought the number up to thirteen.

By now stories about the troubles at the home had begun to filter out. Reporter William R. Benjamin made a follow-up visit on May 9, but they knew he was coming and Mrs. Ramscar was waiting at the door to give him a tour. The smell was still strong, though not as bad as before. In the dining room, previously suffocating, two women were serving a plentiful dinner of corned beef, stew, vegetables, bread, and hominy to fifteen children, aged two to seven years old, who seemed reasonably clean and healthy. It was all going well until they got to the nursery. Mrs. Ramscar was surprisingly candid as they stood over a sick child who, it would come out later, was being tended to by the home's scrub woman. He won't survive, Mrs. Ramscar told Benjamin, and sure enough, Ludwig Norman, aged five months and seven days, died the very next day of scrofula, a form of tuberculosis. The number of dead children was now fourteen.

The NYSPCC had been hearing complaints about the Old Gentlemen's Unsectarian Home for some time, but they were never able to gather enough evidence for an investigation or trial. Due to the escalation of complaints and the discovery of John Hamill, Elbridge T. Gerry was able to marshal his forces and connections. On May 18, he entered the Unsectarian Home with Benjamin and Edward H. Janes, the Assistant Sanitary Superintendent of the Board of Health. (The NYSPCC had very quickly become a powerful advocate for children, with a telegraph link to police headquarters; the New York District Attorney often authorized them to represent the city in court.)

They were met by William H. Ramscar. Before moving to New York to reinvent himself as a philanthropist, Ramscar had worked as a hardware and junk dealer in Philadelphia. "Business was growing dull and it is natural for business men to make changes some times," he later explained with a cavalier air, unaware that his career path would eventually lead to a cell in the Penitentiary on Blackwell's Island. Ramscar's initial foray into humanitarianism began in 1873, the first year of the Great Depression, when he organized a society located on Thirty-Ninth Street to distribute food to the poor, feeding from 200 to 450 people daily. Then came the Peabody Home, in 1874, which took in poor old ladies. Ramscar resigned from the Peabody in 1876, although others would later claim he was paid to leave.

Almost immediately after his exit, Ramscar established the Old Gentlemen's Unsectarian Home. The Unsectarian Home lost its state charter in 1880, after an investigation by Josephine Shaw Lowell and others from the State Board of Charities ended by declaring Ramscar unfit to run the institution. Ramscar simply moved the home to a new location at Mott Avenue and 165th the following year, and continued operations as if nothing had happened. But now the home took in children as well as old men.

Forty-two children, aged six days to fourteen years old, were housed in the home when Gerry, Benjamin, and Janes stepped inside to conduct their investigation. On every floor and in every part of the house they were hit with "the same sickening smell to be found in children's institutions" that had not been kept clean. In the cellar they found perhaps the biggest reason for the pervasive odor—a water closet unconnected to water and lacking any means for flushing. It sat at the end of a dark, blind hallway, completely unventilated, allowing for a continual, noxious buildup of gas. Whenever the children and the old men needed to use the bathroom they had to walk downstairs from the dormitories on the first, second, and third floors to the cellar, then through the unlit passage to the closet, or they could head outside to a facility in the yard. There was another water closet on the second floor, but apparently only the Ramscars were permitted to use it. Also in the cellar, along with the malodorous water closet, were bins for storing food, the kitchen, and the tiny laundry room that Officer Fitzpatrick had climbed into two months before, and which was still being used by four people as a bedroom.

Upstairs, the dining room was clean and the twenty children they found there appeared in acceptable condition. The dormitories were also all in good order. From Edward H. Janes's point of view, the home's biggest problem was a lack of proper help. For all those children, and the men on the upper floors, there was one nurse, one scrub woman, a laundress, and a cook, and, despite the presence of infants, no wet nurses. Hire additional help and replace the water closet, Janes concluded, and the home could be made suitable for children. The three men left.

But hidden away upstairs during the tour through the premises, a six-year-old girl named Bessie Slocum was on her deathbed. She'd been placed in the home by her mother on March 14, the day before Officer Fitzpatrick's climb through the basement window. Janes had specifically asked Ramscar if there were any other sick children on the premises. "No," Ramscar had lied. Two days later Bessie was dead; the last child to die in the Old Gentlemen's Unsectarian Home.

Afterwards, Ramscar sent a note to Annie Slocum, Bessie's mother, but she was no longer living at the address she had given. This presented them with an additional problem. Bessie's younger brother Alfred was still in their care.

A few hours after Bessie died, an investigator came to the home to collect a complete list of all the children who died while in their care. Bessie's name was not on it. When asked later why they didn't let the investigator know that Bessie had also just died, Ramscar blithely answered, "He never asked."

Edward P. Jenkins, of the NYSPCC, went to the Home two days later expecting to meet Edward H. Janes. While he waited, he noted that the stench had grown worse and that the children were filthy. Do you like it here? he asked a little boy passing by. "No, this is a nasty, dirty place." Janes never showed up, and Jenkins left.

The following day, Benjamin Many, one of the older men from the top floor, put Bessie's body in a wagon and drove her to the morgue. Many was accustomed to doing errands for Ramscar, like begging the local grocers and bakeries for food for the home, for which he was paid $1 a week. Annie Slocum finally learned of her daughter's death the day after Bessie's body was taken away, when she came to the home to look in on her. (Mrs. Slocum had just recently moved and planned to let them know her new address during that visit.) Arrangements were made for Bessie to be buried the next morning at St. Michael's Cemetery in Astoria, in the area they had designated for the poor. Annie took her remaining child home.

An inquest was convened in June. Coroner John Brady focused primarily on the death of Bessie Slocum, and less on the fourteen infants who had died between January 2 and May 10. Lowering infant mortality was a challenge for everyone, and the city was also struggling to keep the infants in its care alive. Of the 494 children who died in the Foundling Asylum of the Sisters of Charity that year (roughly a third of the total population of children in the institution), 85.6 percent were under a year old.

None of the various doctors who were called to testify remembered seeing John Hamill. That's because he wasn't seen by a doctor, and had instead been examined by one of the old men on the third floor. That was after Ellen McMasters, the cook, had been asked to see to him and had refused. She was not heartless, just overworked. The children were supposed to get weekly baths, but it was usually just her doing the bathing, and in the two months she had been there, the children in the institution had been bathed only twice. So Mr. Roberts was prevailed upon to pitch in and look over the Hamill boy. Twenty minutes later, Roberts proclaimed him free of vermin, and aside from a rash, he thought he seemed all right. Mr. Roberts, however, had since died and could not be called upon to testify.

Ramscar would later argue that John Hamill had only been in their care for one day, so they could not possibly be responsible for what was obviously a long-term condition. That was a reasonable point, but how could they have missed the fact that his leg was falling off? When asked about the general carelessness in washing and cleaning the children and their clothes, Ramscar answered, "I do not consider that there was any carelessness, we can not always be responsible for what nurses do." To which Brady hotly responded, "Do you thoroughly understand a man employing help, a man having charge of any place is held responsible?"

Everyone testified that Bessie Slocum had been sick for months, except her mother, who had visited her on the Tuesday before she died. According to Mrs. Slocum, "when I saw her that day I never recollect her feeling so happy in my life, she looked to be in perfect health. She had had a cold but she got over it." Annie had asked her daughter if she wanted to go home, and Bessie answered, "No mama, I like to stay here I am so happy." Perhaps Mrs. Slocum was tormented with guilt for having left her sick daughter in a place that would ultimately kill her, and had to tell herself that the home and Bessie had been just fine.

On June 5, the coroner's jury provided their verdict. They found that

> Bessie Slocum died of pneumonia, we also find that she did not have the proper and timely assistance of a physician, through the neglect of the management of the institution.
>
> As to the death of the other children and the causes which led to their deaths we find that the general uncleanliness of the institution, and the presence of foul and impure air, the want of sufficient and experienced nurses and the gross negligence and incompetency of management contributed to the death of these children.
>
> As to who is responsible for the deaths we believe that owing to the alarming death rate recorded according to the testimony given the cause was chiefly through the neglect and incompetency of the general management and service of the institution. We further find from the evidence given that the institution is unworthy of existence and undeserving of public confidence and that it would be in the interest of humanity that the institution be abolished. Further that the management is deserving of special censure on account of the manner of conducting the institution.

Ramscar was promptly arrested and sent to the Tombs, the city jail in lower Manhattan. His lawyer argued that as he was now charged with a crime, Ramscar was entitled to a hearing before a police justice. A coroner was not a magistrate. On June 16 Ramscar appeared before Justice Butler Bixby at the Jefferson Market Courthouse. Bixby only heard the testimony of witnesses like Ellen McMasters, who'd been promoted the month before and who now testified that the children were well fed and cared for, and were sent off to school every day bright, clean, and happy. He did not hear from anyone who had been critical of the conditions. Bixby said he could therefore find no proof of neglect and ordered Ramscar discharged, although the order to remove all the children from the home remained in force. According to the *New-York Tribune*, as Edward F. Jenkins led the children away, Ramscar looked on "smilingly" and talked about the new home he planned to establish for "adult incurables." Brady, the coroner, who was apoplectic, would protest that even drunks got ten days on the Island.

Two years later, Ramscar was running an institution called the Home for Children and Seminary for Girls in a single-family house at 153rd Street and St. Nicholas Avenue. He'd recently taken to wearing clothes with a decidedly "clerical cut." While not a minister of the gospel, he would later explain, he wore outfits that looked like that of a clergyman because he was "a minister outside of the church," and felt entitled to look the part. In place of old men, Ramscar was now sending the children in his care out in a wagon two or three times a week to beg the local butchers, bakers, and grocers for food. This was against the law. The NYSPCC investigated, and Ramscar was arrested on July 9, 1884, and tried in the Court of General Sessions in November, before Recorder Frederick Smyth. The jury found him guilty, but recommended mercy. Ramscar must have put on a convincing show. Smyth sentenced him to one month in the Tombs and a fine of $100.

By 1886 the Old Gentlemen's Unsectarian Home was back in business, this time at Tenth Avenue and 175th Street. Complaints about the care of children once again started flowing into the NYSPCC, and the home was investigated by a grand jury. Although the investigators came back with glowing reviews—one juror said he'd be "delighted if my own children were as healthy, as fair, as rosy-cheeked, as chubby"—it came out that the home did not currently have a permit to board children.

Ramscar applied to the Board of Health for the necessary permit, but Elbridge T. Gerry did everything he could to oppose the application, including writing to the board to point out, among other things, that Ramscar was currently boarding children, so he was already guilty of a misdemeanor. While the board considered his application, Ramscar wrote Gerry, warning him, "This Institution has suffered great losses in consequence of the numerous malicious attacks made upon it by you, and especially on account of your vile and inhuman accusations . . . I deem it wise to respectfully ask you to retract through the public press before Saturday next . . . otherwise legal processing will be instituted against you." The Board of Health ultimately decided to refuse to grant the permit, and the parents were notified to remove their children. The next year Ramscar sued Gerry for libel. His complaint was dismissed.

If nothing else, Ramscar was a rebounder. A year later, in a Washington Heights mansion overlooking the Hudson River, he established the National Unsectarian Home for Worthy, Aged and Destitute People and Incurables, Irrespective of Creed or Nationality. But Ramscar didn't manage to stay out of trouble long. When John Laverty visited the home in 1889 to see if this was a place where he could live, Ramscar showed him one of the best rooms in the estate. Laverty put down money to cover three months. After a few nights, Ramscar told him he had to move to the attic.

It was a bait-and-switch tactic he'd used before. When one man looked into putting his father-in-law in the home, he'd been told there were two prices: $2 a week, where you ate what you could get, or $3 a week for the best food and the nicest rooms. The food was the same for all, of course; it was gathered by employing the aforementioned begging wagon from 1884, and was often so putrid the men fell sick. During the three months the man's father-in-law was there at the $3 rate, he'd been allowed one bath, and for that he was taken to a barn and hosed down. In a room no better than any other, he slept on a cot that had originally been bought for Ramscar's children's home and wasn't long enough for him to stretch out his legs.

John Laverty was a tough seventy-two-year-old, and when he was told to move to the attic, he refused. Ramscar beat him with a bat. Laverty ran out into the street and found a police officer who took him to a hospital. He got four stitches for a gash in his head, and Ramscar was arrested.

At the trial, which was postponed when Ramscar's wife passed away, Ramscar claimed self-defense. He said Laverty had been drinking and attacked him. The doctor who treated Laverty and the officer who took him to the hospital testified that they saw no signs of intoxication.

While court had been adjourned out of respect for Mrs. Ramscar's demise, Recorder Smyth received a letter from a former employee of the home. The man told a revolting story of what life was truly like for the old men inside, which confirmed much of what they'd heard and was in keeping with Ramscar's history. The man had been asked to change the bed sheets for Colonel Benton, a retired military man and a graduate of West Point. He found Benton soiled with excrement from his "hips to his knees," and the mattress "saturated with urine." On closer inspection he realized that the mattress was "literally alive with small white worms." There were no bathing facilities at the home, he went on, and there were also no "disinfectants or any medical appliances" of any kind. In order to discourage the inmates, many of whom were near-paupers, from requesting medical attention, they were charged $2 each time a doctor came to see them. The men were "mostly old, decrepit people, poor," the former employee wrote, and "as much at the mercy of one man as the subjects of the Russian despot."

Ramscar was found guilty on December 18. Before the sentence was pronounced, he was given a chance to speak. He cited what he saw as all his previous good works, and then pointed to his new wife, whom he'd married two weeks after his first wife had died. "In consideration of my service to the community restore me to that weeping wife, that noble young lady of refined and brilliant qualities who has joined with me in caring for the poor and unfortunate."

Smyth declined. For having "made a cruel and unprovoked assault upon a feeble old man," he began, "I can see no reason why I should not impose the extreme penalty of the law under your conviction." Fifteen children died while in his care and there had been no repercussions. But now he was going to spend a year in the Penitentiary on Blackwell's Island. He was admitted on Christmas Eve.

Five years (one of them in the Penitentiary) and two more failed institutions later—the National Unsectarian Home, where he was arrested again for beating up another inmate, and the Cornwall Retreat, "a non-sectarian institution for old and feeble-minded people," which never attracted enough funding to open its doors—Ramscar was able to get the new National Non-Sectarian Home for Old Ladies off the ground. "We are very fond of the ladies," his wife was quoted as saying, "and my husband and I find them much easier to manage than old men, who are apt to be ungrateful and quarrelsome, while children are a great responsibility." A reporter visiting the rooms wrote, "As we climbed the stairs the stench of filth and disease grew stronger," and the one room he saw "was as vile a little hole as can be imagined."

Ramscar was arrested again in 1903, when he was found begging in the streets. It was for his Cornwall Retreat, he told the judge before being sent back to Blackwell's Island to serve a six-month sentence in the Workhouse for vagrancy. He was jailed again in 1910, this time for not paying wages to the employees of his latest institution, the Margaret Jane Non-Sectarian Home for Aged Indigent People and Incurables From All States. Four years later he died there, on May 22, 1914, at age eighty. Due to his reduced circumstances, he was laid to rest in St. Michael's Cemetery, the same cemetery where six-year-old Bessie Slocum was buried all those years before.

REVEREND EDWARD COWLEY

The Shepherd's Fold
Sentenced to the Penitentiary February 20, 1880

⬦

O N THE DAY after Christmas, 1879, a six-year-old boy named Louis Victor was brought to St. Luke's Hospital in upper Manhattan from a charitable institution called the Shepherd's Fold. Louis had been diagnosed with rickets and he wasn't getting any better, even though his caretakers later insisted that they'd carefully followed the treatment prescribed. Dr. John Ridlon, a resident, was in charge that night. Louis was severely emaciated and Dr. Ridlon questioned Sophia Cowley, the woman who'd brought Louis in. What was he fed? Mrs. Cowley described his diet as "farinaceous," by which she meant not a lot of meat. Ridlon wanted specifics. "What did he have for breakfast?" he asked. "Oatmeal and milk." And lunch? At this point Mrs. Cowley turned to Bessie Lawrence, the girl who had accompanied them. "What do you have?" she asked the girl. Mrs. Cowley, the doctor realized, didn't know.

Ridlon later described Louis as "simply skin and bones; there was no signs of any fat or muscular development. . . . He was very pale; on the tarsus of his left foot there was an ulcer as large as a quarter dollar. . . . There was a small bed-sore over the left hip bone, and two or three small abrasions along the spinal column where the hips stuck out. . . . He made, during the time I was examining him in the office in the presence of Mrs.

Cowley, no cry, or noise whatever, and after he was taken to the ward he continually cried for food, especially for meat." In the doctor's opinion he was facing an advanced case of starvation.

Ridlon contacted the New York Society for the Prevention of Cruelty to Children on January 6, 1880, and asked them to come have a look at the boy. As it happened, the Society already had their eye on the Reverend Edward Cowley, the Superintendent of the Shepherd's Fold, and they'd been waiting for just such a message.

THE SHEPHERD'S FOLD evolved out of Cowley's history as a missionary on Blackwell's Island, when more than half the children admitted to the Almshouse every year died. Cowley believed if he could get a group of wealthy, influential society ladies to regularly visit the nurseries, mortality rates would go down. Perhaps he thought the workers on the Island would realize they had to put on a good show. The ladies came and Cowley's instincts proved correct, but the results were modest. The most effective long-term answer, Cowley felt, would be to bypass the Island altogether. In 1867, Cowley, the ladies, and others, established the Shepherd's Fold as an alternative place to take in abandoned children. The city quickly incorporated the Fold the following year. Factions soon developed among the institution's board, however, and in 1869 everyone in Cowley's camp left to assume control of another institution Cowley had helped to organize, the Children's Fold, which was incorporated in 1871—Cowley's last full year as a Blackwell's Island missionary. Afterwards, the Shepherd's Fold began a slow decline, and by 1874 operations had ceased entirely.

The first complaint about the Children's Fold came into the NYSPCC in January, 1875, when the Society was in its first year of operation. The situation didn't sound particularly dire. Cowley had kicked a child, they were told. A year later, a former matron at the now-defunct Shepherd's Fold said that Cowley was starving the children over at the Children's Fold. Before the year was out they'd receive two more complaints of starvation. Finally, a parent contacted the State Board of Charities, and from the fall of 1876 to January 1877, Josephine Shaw Lowell, Theodore Roosevelt, and Henry L. Hoquet formed a committee and began a secret investigation of the Children's Fold.

The committee members spoke to current and former employers, but the most damning reports came from children themselves. News of the investigation leaked out and all the papers published the most lurid details. Cowley often beat them with a shoe or a slipper, whichever was nearer, the children said, and sometimes he used a whip. Jennie Mills, who was eighteen years old and had been with Cowley since she was ten, said on one occasion he hit her brother with a shoe and made his head bleed. Mills also told them that Cowley punished Fannie McCurdy so often that whenever he approached, "she would kneel to him in the most abject manner." "Lay it on her good," Cowley was reported to have said to his wife as she beat boarder Kate McCurdy for a half an hour with a brush. When Mrs. Cowley tired, Cowley took over and continued the attack.

It was true that he punished the children, Cowley conceded, but "only in a fatherly way, and Jennie must be mistaken about my using extreme cruelty." A *New-York Tribune* reporter brought Jennie Mills and Cowley together. Cowley fully expected Mills to recant when confronted, and seemed genuinely shocked when she insisted she wasn't exaggerating. The next day, in a brief editorial, the *Tribune* would write, "The new system of using shoes and whips on children 'in a fatherly way' has not proved a gigantic success."

Josephine Shaw Lowell declared Cowley "utterly unfit to manage any charitable institution," and Cowley was allowed to resign in February 1877, although he remained a member of the board of the Children's Fold.

Cowley continued to see himself as the injured party. He wrote the State Board of Charities committee to insist that there were people who wished to ruin him, and while he had not handled his opposition wisely, he admitted, he was innocent of the charges against him. Cowley also wrote a letter to editor of the *New York Herald*, addressing each accusation. The incident Jennie Mills described, for instance, was not witnessed by her and could not be corroborated by anyone, including her brother, and Kate McCurdy denied the story about being beaten with a brush.

If there really were forces working against him, they may have been coming from Cowley himself. He had such poor anger management and people skills that it wasn't just the children who wanted him to go away. James Pott, one of the original founders of the Children's Fold, said that while the accounts of cruelty had been exaggerated, and they happened a long time ago, Cowley nonetheless had an "ungovernable temper, which led him to exceed the bounds of reason at times." When Elias J. Pattison, another Children's Fold founder, was questioned about Cowley's resignation, he didn't even mention the abuse until asked specifically in a follow-up question. Instead, Pattison said they asked him to resign because they "could not stand him any longer."

"It was difficult to get rid of this man," Pattison complained. "He was not one of those people who could be easily suppressed, and even when you did effect his removal you could not tell when or where you would find him next."

Where Cowley ended up next was right back at the Shepherd's Fold. A month after resigning from the Children's Fold, eight of the original founders formed a new Board of Trustees and elected Rev. Cowley to revive and manage the dormant Shepherd's Fold.

The founders who were not included in this maneuver formed their own Board of Trustees to take over the Shepherd's Fold, and elected the Reverend Thomas McClure Peters to head their board. Peters was the Rector of St. Michael's Protestant Episcopal Church, which had established the cemetery for the poor in Astoria, where some of the dead from Blackwell's were buried. He was also known for having organized another charitable institution for children, the Sheltering Arms, and he was the one who'd been asked to take Cowley's place as the President of the Executive Committee of the Children's Fold after Cowley had been removed due to the State Charities Aid Association report.

What's more, Rev. Peters was one of the earliest members of the growing

group of people who'd been alienated by Cowley's sometimes erratic behavior. In 1871, while Cowley was a missionary on Blackwell's Island, Rev.
Peters was the chairman of the Committee of Direction for the New York
Protestant Episcopal Mission Society, the group that oversaw the Episcopal
mission on Blackwell's Island. Cowley had written Peters to tell him that
the commissioners of the Department of Public Charities and Correction
were denying him the use of the Island Chapel. Go back to the commissioners and demand your rights, Peters instructed him. Later, a committee including Peters formed to aid Cowley, and the committee asked the
commissioners to restore all the rights and privileges the Episcopal Mission Society had previously enjoyed as missionaries on Blackwell's Island.

Sometime in April, without a word to the Board, Cowley abruptly left
his mission on Blackwell's Island. Peters was assigned to find out why. Unable to get a clear explanation out of Cowley, the frustrated committee met
with the commissioners themselves, where they were told that not only had
"Mr. Cowley left the Island of his own will and pleasure . . . he had been
very remiss in his attendance" in some areas on the Island. (A newspaper
would later report that Cowley refused to enter the smallpox hospital, but
the Episcopal Mission Society's minutes offer no specifics.)

The Board quickly convened an emergency evening meeting in the
home of the bishop, where it was decided to officially terminate Cowley's
engagement as a missionary. Three weeks later, Dr. Peters nominated Rev.
French as Cowley's replacement. The motion was carried and French was
appointed with a salary of $2,000 a year. The committee again met with
Cowley to hear why he had left the Island, but he was no more forthcoming
than he had been the last time. The minutes say only that Peters met with
him, "but owing to some feelings on the part of Mr. Cowley, the meeting
was in no way satisfactory."

Six years later, Cowley and Peters were head to head once again, this
time over who had the right to run the Shepherd's Fold. Peters had since
grown into a powerful and well-connected adversary, who boasted a former mayor on his board, while Cowley seemed to have spent the same time

driving still more people away. At issue was $5,000 that the state comptroller had been authorized to pay to the Shepherd's Fold yearly. When Cowley resumed control of the Shepherd's Fold they immediately applied for two years' back annuity. The comptroller now had two sets of officers asking for the money, and told them the money would be withheld until the courts decided which board was entitled to it.

The court initially ruled in favor of Cowley in 1879. The Peters faction immediately appealed, and a judge in the general term of the Supreme Court reversed the earlier decision, ordering a new trial. The father of Louis Victor, the little boy who had shown up ill at St. Luke's, had delivered his son to the Shepherd's Fold in the midst of this struggle for control, and after a few months of regular visits the father was never seen again. When Sophia Cowley brought Louis to St. Luke's Hospital three months after the court's decision, the attorney general had not yet taken any action. Cowley had been running the Shepherd's Fold without the state funds, and with a daily average of twenty-five orphans in their care.

Based on intelligence from Dr. Ridlon, and an incriminating photograph of Louis Victor looking like a tiny skeleton, Elbridge Gerry and the NYSPCC were able to get a court order to remove the remaining children from the Fold. On January 17, six coaches pulled up in front of the Fold's four-story brownstone at 157 E. Sixtieth Street. Twenty-four children were extracted and taken straight to a restaurant for lunch, where they pounced on everything put in front of them. Although much was written in the papers about how ravenously they fed, it came out later that the children were taken from the Fold just before their next meal, when they would have been hungry in any case. Given that oatmeal was their usual meal, it's no wonder they devoured what must have seemed an almost impossibly sumptuous feast of roast beef, stuffed veal, and piles of "dainties." From the restaurant, the children were marched into court, where they made a captivating *King and I*–like procession, some children walking, with younger ones carried by employees of the NYSPCC. All court business stopped while everyone watched their entrance.

On that first day they heard initial testimony from the Cowleys, Elbridge Gerry, and the sister-in-law of Louis Victor's father. The proceedings were then adjourned for a week so Cowley's lawyers could prepare his defense. When Cowley was indicted a couple of weeks later, the case was moved to the Court of General Session under Recorder Frederick Smyth, the same judge who would later sit on the trials of William Ramscar. Bail was set too high for Cowley, and until his friends raised the money a week later, like everyone else under indictment, Cowley was sent to the Tombs and taken to court each day handcuffed to his fellow prisoners, marched through the prison yard, and piled into the Black Maria.

The newspapers made much of the wealthy women packed into the courtroom each day, who "sat four deep in the seats allotted to extra jurymen, filled every inch of space in the witness box, and invaded the enclosure occupied" by the district attorney and his assistant. During recess, "the Cowley coterie . . . ate lunch, cracked nuts, and enjoyed themselves immensely."

Over the next month, a sensational story emerged. One father said he put his son Harry into the Fold, and he came out starving, unable to walk, his hair thick with vermin. "There was a continuous sore from one corner of his mouth to the other. The right side of the lower lip was eaten in," making a hole so big you could fit "a small pipe stem" through it. The principal of a nearby public school said that at different times seven Fold children attended her school, often showing up dressed in dirty clothes, with "sore eyes," ringworm, vermin, and, above all, hungry. She sometimes caught them stealing food from their fellow students and teachers, and snatching discarded bits of bread and apple cores from the street.

On January 24, fifteen-year-old Emma Bowen took the stand. She'd been with Cowley and his wife Sophia since she was two, when she was indentured to them from the Department of Public Charities and Correction. Also indentured that year were Emma Hawes and Charles Underhill, who were both two years old, and John Campbell, who was three. Like Mary Ellen, all the indenture terms in the children's contracts were crossed out and replaced with terms describing an adoption. The children lived with the Cowleys in Charity Hospital on Blackwell's Island until Cowley left his mission in 1872, and they stayed with the Cowleys from Fold to Fold. It gives the impression that they were all a family, but as the children had grown older, they evolved into "the help."

There were no servants or workers at the Shepherd's Fold by the time Sophia Cowley took Louis Victor to the hospital. Instead, every morning Emma Bowen, Emma Hawes—who was now called Lillie—and other girls, like Fanny McCurdy, who'd been placed there by her father in 1871, got up out of bed at five o'clock to begin the work of the institution. After feeding breakfast to all the children, which was generally bread, Indian meal mush, and condensed milk (one part milk to eighteen parts water), they would spend the rest of their day cleaning, scrubbing, and doing laundry. The girls would work until nine at night, with one hour to themselves before bedtime. The boys worked outside and did most of the begging, which is how much of the food for the children was acquired.

However, aside from the begging, these revelations described the standard operating procedure inside many charitable institutions in the city. Older children frequently were responsible for day-to-day chores. If this had been all the prosecution had, there wouldn't be much of a case. But Emma testified that Cowley on various occasions hit, kicked, and whipped her with a cat of nine tails. "Once before he knocked me down on the floor with his clenched fist and then stamped upon me; he made bruises on my legs, and as I lay down he also beat me with his fist." On another occasion Cowley locked her up in the attic for a week, where she was fed only bread and water. While the Cowleys were vehemently defending the benefits of a vegetarian diet for the children, Emma talked about the bountiful dinners of steaks, chops, and cakes that were typically served to the Cowleys.

Fanny McCurdy, described by one newspaper as tall and cross-eyed, said that one Sunday after church, Cowley "hit me across the back with a poker. Charley Fox [formerly named Charles Underhill] had told him something about me. Without giving me time to answer he took the poker and hit me with it as hard as he could on the shoulder. . . . My shoulder was swollen by the blow, and the swelling lasted several days." Another time, he hit her because she hadn't "ironed his shirts right."

This was certainly very damaging if true, but Cowley was on trial for his treatment of Louis Victor. It all came down to this: Did Cowley respond appropriately to Louis's medical issues, and did he make sure Louis was adequately fed?

When Louis first started showing symptoms the previous summer, the Cowleys took him to Dr. Walker A. Hawes, the Fold's attending physician. Hawes diagnosed Louis with rickets. It was not an uncommon childhood affliction among the poor, although the causes were not understood at the time. They had begun to realize it had something to do with sunlight and diet, and Hawes's prescription included increasing Louis's time outdoors in the fresh air and lots of food. The Cowleys followed Hawes's instructions and initially Louis rallied. But he fell sick again that October, and when Dr. Hawes returned to the Fold, Louis was now diarrhetic and looked emaciated. This was due to his lack of digestive powers, Hawes told them, which was also a symptom of rickets. He prescribed cod-liver oil, iron, and more food, sunlight and exercise. Despite their efforts, Louis failed to recover this time, and Mrs. Cowley brought him to the hospital.

Dr. Hawes was forty years old when he took the stand in 1880. He'd been practicing medicine since 1866, and his background included one year as an assistant to the Chair of Diseases of Children at the New York Polyclinic Medical School and Hospital, and two years as a visiting physician to the Almshouse and Workhouse hospitals. He verified that he saw Louis four times, twice at the Fold and twice in his office, and that he had diagnosed Louis with rickets. A rickets diagnosis was perfectly reasonable. Called a "disease of malnutrition" by doctors in the nineteenth century, it appeared to be due to either insufficient feeding, or some other cause which impeded digestion. Dr. Hawes was prescribing what would later be found as the most effective possible treatment for rickets—sunlight and cod-liver oil, precisely because exposure to sunlight and cod-liver oil are excellent sources of vitamin D.

But the prosecution called four doctors with overwhelmingly more impressive resumes, including Dr. Abraham Jacobi, who was then teaching medicine at Columbia University, and would go on to establish a Department of Pediatrics at Mt. Sinai, the first of its kind; Dr. Frank Hastings Hamilton, a distinguished physician who would be brought to Washington, D.C., the following year to tend to President James Garfield after he'd been shot; and Dr. Edward C. Spitzka, who was actually better known for his work in psychiatry (he testified later that year at the hearing of the State Committee on Insanity, criticizing the doctors at Blackwell's Lunatic Asylum). It was a formidable lineup, and each doctor dismissed the diagnosis of rickets, arguing that all of Louis's symptoms were due to starvation.

Cowley's lawyer pointed out that Spitzka saw Louis on January 30, after he'd been in the hospital for a month. If Louis was still emaciated after being in their care for a month, the hospital was having just as much trouble treating him as the Cowleys.

Spitzka was recalled. Yes, Louis was still thin at the end of the month, but he was looking better than he had when the condemnatory photograph was taken. "I am satisfied that there never was the slightest ground for supposing that the child had suffered from rickets; the disease always leaves permanent traces, and there were none present."

The children's testimony was conflicting. One girl said she never saw Mrs. Cowley give Louis iron or cod-liver oil. Another said she did. There was a lot of disagreement about what he was fed, but more than one witness testified that they saw Louis being given fruit, tomatoes, meat, and eggs.

One member of Cowley's legal team, an ex-judge named William Fullerton, made some strong points. "The fact was," he told the court, "a physician told Mr. Cowley that Louis Victor was suffering from rickets. Whether it was so or not, he believed it." Further, if the diet was so dangerously inadequate, why weren't all the children in the hospital? In the last two years the only child who'd become ill while in Cowley's care was

Louis. "That fact speaks more loudly than the medical testimony about the nutrition of the food." In the past twelve years, Cowley had overseen the care of 600 children, and only three had died. While any number of deaths sounds bad, compared to every other institution at the time, especially the Department of Public Charities and Correction, Cowley's track record was excellent. Fullerton also pointed out that the prosecution had not produced Louis Victor to show that he was truly doing any better. "How far has he advanced in strength since he has been in the hospital?"

Cowley's legal team was hampered by the fact that the children from the Fold had been taken to an undisclosed location and while they were made available to the prosecution team, they were never made available to the defense, except when they were cross-examined in court. It also didn't help that the press had already decided the case against Cowley. But in the end, Cowley's lawyers put up a terrible defense. The witnesses they brought forward were few and unconvincing. District Attorney Benjamin K. Phelps, on the other hand, brought in the big guns, who were not only more compelling, they were entertaining. Dr. James W. Ranney testified that, of the twenty-four children he examined, only three were strong and healthy, especially the girl who worked in the kitchen, he joked, prompting laughter throughout the courtroom. The defense compounded their loss in that moment by not even bothering to cross-examine him. Cowley's side seemed utterly unprepared to take on the much stronger and better prepared prosecution.

In his closing argument, Phelps pressed an obvious advantage by reminding the jury that only one member of the original board of the Shepherd's Fold had shown up to speak on Cowley's behalf and that was his brother. "Why have these men not rallied around their Secretary?" Where was anyone who knew his work of nine years on Blackwell's Island?

It took the jury only eighteen minutes to find Cowley guilty. Recorder Smyth would say, "In my judgment they could not arrive at any other conclusion." The only thing left to do was sentence him.

A contemporary of Smyth's said that, from the bench, Smyth came off "as a veritable sphinx—impassive, stern and uncompromising." But he was also famous for pronouncing his sentences gently, and with compassion. Smyth turned and faced Cowley. "I have no desire to add anything to the pain you must feel at this moment, by any remarks I might make," he said to the defeated priest. "I will end by passing on you the sentence that the law demands."

Smyth sentenced Cowley to one year in the Penitentiary and an additional fine of $250. Cowley would appeal and lose.

The Nation published an editorial criticizing the NYSPCC and the Department of Public Charities and Correction. The "treatment of Cowley before trial has been a somewhat painful spectacle to the lovers of fair play." Particularly, "the permission given to his fellow-prisoners in the Tombs to mock and jeer at him out of their cells was a great outrage." The editors agreed that the children should have been cared for better, "but the evidence of children, like that of grown people, needs sifting, and there was from the beginning a possibility that Cowley had been led into his offense, partly at least, by undertaking to support more children than he had the money for, and not wholly cruelty and greed."

Later, some of the children who testified against him would recant. "I wouldn't have said as much as I did against him," Fanny McCurdy confessed, "if I hadn't been put up to it. I don't recollect what I said . . . I was so frightened. . . . It is too late to alter it now—I must stick to it." She also admitted to being resentful about all the work she was made to do at the Fold. She thought she should have been paid.

When the time came to take Cowley to the Island he broke down. "This is hard, very hard," he said to the police who entered his cell to escort him to the dock. Then he bent his head down and sobbed, while trying to hide his face with his hands. He'd boarded the steamboat *Minnahanonck* (the early Indian name for Blackwell's Island) thousands of times as a missionary. But to now come aboard as a prisoner, where he was met by Captain Steele, who knew him from the old days—it was so mortifying Cowley didn't know where to look. The old captain took pity on the priest and shook his hand.

Warden John Fox also tried to extend to him every possible professional courtesy. Cowley kept hoping for a stay of his sentence. This was all a horrible miscarriage of justice that someone would right. Any minute now. Fox waited politely for three-quarters of an hour.

But the time came for Cowley to confront the unavoidably humiliating process of admission. That year, 1,958 people were received by the Penitentiary, only ten of whom were sent there for cruelty to children, which was still a new crime. Cowley was brought into the reception room and added to their log books. The entry for Cowley reads: "Committed February 20; received March 2; Cowley, Edward: 52; one year, $250 fine, or 250 days; 5 feet 2 1/2 inches; 137 pounds, crime, cruelty to a child; hair gray, eyes gray, dark complexioned: England; 45 year in United states; married; educated, Protestant minister."

From there, Cowley was made to sit in a barber chair, where his hair was cut and his carefully tended beard was completely shaved away. He was then stripped naked and put in one of three bathtubs pushed up against the wall, and publicly scrubbed. Afterwards he was issued his suit of stripes and assigned to the shoe shop, a relatively easy detail. The keeper was instructed to punish anyone who taunted or insulted Cowley.

There may have been a few prisoners there who knew him from before, and were dying to give back a little of what Cowley was said to have given them. According to one colorful newspaper account, while a missionary on the Island, Cowley had "ordered prisoners into the dark cell for coughing during service." It seems hard to believe he could be so cruel and petty, but toward the end of that year District Attorney Benjamin K. Phelps fell ill and he died on December 30, nine days after his wife, who'd died on December 21. In a letter to Elbridge Gerry, Cowley wrote that "his ailing and death, and that of his wife, are the fullest vindication that I could desire." One can certainly understand it if Cowley felt little sympathy for the D.A., but his wife? It betrays such a mean streak that at least some of the accusations against him seem more plausible. In any case, Cowley would now be sitting before the same pulpit, it was gleefully reported, from which he had once stood behind to preach to those prisoners all those years ago.

Aside from being assigned to the shoe shop instead of a chain gang breaking rocks, Cowley's time on the Island does not appear to be any different from any other prisoners. It was certainly possible to bribe yourself into an easier stay. Emma Goldman, who spent ten months in prison from October 1893 to August 1894, wrote about the head matron of the women's side of the Penitentiary, Isabella De Graff. Although she greeted Goldman warmly, and treated her well during her time there (without any prompting or bribe from Goldman), De Graff was a nightmare to the rest of the prisoners in her care, according to Goldman, unless you paid her off. "The greatest pleasure of the head matron is to torment and plague both her assistant and the prisoners. Nothing satisfies her, nothing pleases her."

De Graff once assigned a sick, seventy-year-old woman to scrubbing. When the doctor demanded that the woman be sent to the hospital, De Graff insisted that she was faking, and "continued to abuse her until for some reason she suddenly became all sympathy and attention," but it was too late. The woman died a day before her sentence was ended, "legally murdered," according to Goldman.

The Deputy Warden defended his head matron and denied all of Goldman's charges, but later someone quietly solicited testimony about her from former workers and prisoners. A night matron swore that De Graff would extort money and gifts from the prisoners, and they would be rewarded with special privileges if they complied, and punished if they didn't. One prisoner said it cost her $5 to avoid abuse, and others testified that if they didn't come up with anything worthy during their time there De Graff would continue to hound them to send something to her after they got out. Everyone talked about the prisoner who was detailed as De Graff's personal manicurist, and who got decent food, whiskey, and wine, not only as a reward for doing De Graff's nails, but for spying and reporting on her fellow inmates.

There was never much outrage about the conditions at the Penitentiary.

Most people felt that, even more than the inmates of the Workhouse, those sentenced to the Penitentiary were getting what they deserved. Josephine Shaw Lowell, in her 1880 report on all the institutions of the Department of Public Charities and Correction, doesn't even mention it. The people who worked at the Penitentiary, however, repeatedly called attention to the problems there. When Keen was warden he wrote about the crowded conditions, and how the "night is made hideous with the yells and fightings" of the men, crammed in as they were. Katherine B. Davis, the Commissioner of the Department of Correction, called the Penitentiary "vile and inhuman" and the cells "wet, slimy, dark, foul smelling, and unfit for pigs to wallow in." Although Keen and Davis are talking about conditions in 1852 and 1914, respectively, the descriptions would apply to the prison in any year.

There is no evidence Cowley did anything other than serve his sentence stoically. He would have been assigned to a cell unfit for a pig and, like all the other men, he would have marched from place to place in lockstep, without talking, grimly proceeding to meals three times a day, where, like almost everyone else on Blackwell's, he was slowly starved. Improperly feeding someone was a felony, and it was what brought Cowley to the Penitentiary, but no one in the Department of Public Charities and Correction, or the city's Board of Estimate and Apportionment, ever went to prison for the decades-long famine on Blackwell's.

Rev. French once wrote about the Island, "I have often said to myself while going from one scene of suffering to another, 'I could never stand it to live in the midst of this misery.'" How did he stand it when he came across one of his own? It would have been a wretched encounter had it occurred, but perhaps it was one that both men successfully avoided. French was not allowed to visit anyone in their cell. If he saw Cowley at all it would have been at services once a month, or in the hospital, if Cowley had ever ended up there. But Cowley could have stayed away from services and the hospital, if he was lucky. French did write to Cowley on April 8, about a month after he'd been admitted.

My Dear Brother:

At your suggestion I give you my honest judgment of your work on Blackwell's Island during the nine years that you were in charge. That great progress has been made since your departure, is evident; but it is quite as evident that this progress could not have been effected without your previous work. I have often thought, when estimating the present condition of things, of St. Paul's words, "One soweth and another reapeth— one layeth the foundation and another buildeth thereon." A strong foundation was laid by you, and I have done something towards building, which God has prospered . . .

I should feel it to be a great wrong to you, for me to say one word in disparagement of the important part you have had in building up of St. Lazarus' Mission Parish.

Wishing you a speedy release from your bonds, I am, very sincerely,

Your friend and brother in Christ,

W. G. French

That summer, while Cowley was on the Island, the case deciding who controlled the Shepherd's Fold was finally resolved. As Cowley was in prison and no one in his faction appeared on their behalf, Peters and his board were declared the true trustees and managers.

Cowley's term was to end in February 1881, but he was granted a one-month reduction for good behavior, and he left Blackwell's Island for the last time on January 10, 1881.

At the request of both Rev. Cowley and Elbridge Gerry, the Episcopal Church began its own investigation into Cowley's management of the Shepherd's Fold. Gerry wanted to see Cowley defrocked, and Cowley was looking for vindication. The Church's report was published in June, 1881, and it suggests that Cowley might have been his own worst enemy. They found that "the Rev. Edward Cowley had not been conspicuous among his associates for prudence or for winning ways," and instead "displayed a rare aptitude, indeed, for creating alienations and making enemies." But they did not find "anything of a positively criminal character had ever been imputed to Mr. Cowley by those who had long known him, and had shared with him various and serious responsibilities." Despite his poor people skills, his "years of service as a missionary on Blackwell's Island had won and maintained a reputation for kindness and fidelity which survives to this day."

The committee did not whitewash Cowley. What softened their response was the testimony the court had never heard. They spoke to a visitor to the Home for the Friendless, where the children had been taken after being removed from the Fold. The woman spent time with them right after they were admitted, and found "that in all apparent respects they seemed like the children" who were current inmates of the Home for the Friendless, and in no better or worse shape. Additional invoices for food were uncovered that seemed to prove that the children were adequately fed. As far as the mostly vegetarian diet, "good authority affirms, so the committee are told at least, that a healthy child, sufficiently fed on such fare, cannot properly be said to be starved."

They summed up the salient points that Cowley's lawyer had already made. That "there is abundant reliable testimony that the sick child in question was taken or sent by Mr. Cowley to a physician of good standing," and that what the "physician deemed proper remedies in the way of food and medicine were not only prescribed but actually furnished and applied." Finally, that "If it was not a case of rickets the Rev. Edward Cowley cannot fairly be counted criminal" for not treating Louis for "some other and to him unknown disease." There would not be an ecclesiastical trial.

The picture of Louis laying in his hospital bed looking like what might now be described as a victim of a concentration camp could not be ignored. It was inconceivable that any reasonable human being could have allowed his condition to deteriorate to that degree. While Cowley could not be held responsible for the doctor's misdiagnosis, the Church "most emphatically" condemned him for not taking Louis to the hospital until long after it was obvious that the treatments the doctor had suggested were not working.

After his release, over the next two years, Cowley and his brother published several documents in his defense, including an open letter from the Rev. Cowley to Elbridge Gerry. If Gerry really believed terrible things were happening at the Fold, Cowley asked, "Why, in Heaven's name" did he wait three years to act on them? Cowley's letter continued, "At any hour of the day or night you might have obtained an order from any judge of the Supreme Court appointing an officer to examine and make immediate report of the condition of the Shepherd's Fold; and you could probably have got yourself so appointed." The children regularly appeared in church. Had they "appeared starved or bruised or emaciated," many people would have seen, and yet, no one said a word to anyone. And why wasn't he insisting on a specific diet for all children in all asylums, if a proper diet was his big concern? Children were dying at alarming rates in the city institutions; why hadn't he gone after them?

AT THE SAME time Cowley was writing to Gerry, the coroner's investigation into William Ramscar and the death of fifteen children in the Old Gentlemen's Unsectarian Home was underway. Many, including Elbridge Gerry, were quoted making comparisons between Ramscar and Cowley and proclaiming Cowley as the worse of the two. Cowley called such a conclusion "utterly inexplicable and utterly detestable," only adding to Cowley's own conclusion that Gerry's conduct was "in every way unbecoming a man, and revolting to a Christian."

There were actually twenty-five indictments against Cowley for cruelty to twenty-five children, although he only went to trial for Louis Victor. When Cowley started gathering evidence in 1883 for the other twenty-four charges, Gerry asked Recorder Smyth to order a nolle prosequi on all the remaining indictments. A nolle prosequi refers to the decision to not take a case to trial, and Smyth agreed. The reasons for Gerry's request and Smyth's assent to it are not known, but a nolle prosequi is not the same as an acquittal. For Cowley, it meant that he would never have the opportunity prove his innocence. "If true on Jan. 31, 1880, they were equally true

Feb. 1, 1883, and the prosecution should have tried them. But Mr. Gerry prevented that, and so shielded his agents," Cowley wrote bitterly in a statement titled, "Louis Victor: His Sickness and His Cure."

Rev. James L. Maxwell, who took over the Penitentiary mission, later wrote, "Whatever good resolution a discharged prisoner may have formed as to the future, the fact that he is an ex-convict is a stain that it is not easy to efface. When returning to his former friends he is looked upon as a dangerous man. No one wants to employ a 'prison bird,' however earnest his protestations to lead an honest life, even when it is known that with the exception of the one misstep that caused his arrest and conviction, his life has been blameless."

Cowley still clung to the hope that his innocence would one day be established. In 1884, eminent clergymen like Rev. Joseph Hine Rylance, of St. Mark's Church, and Rev. James Mulcahey, of St. Paul's Chapel, signed a petition to look into the conduct of the officers and managers of the New York Society of the Prevention of Cruelty to Children towards Rev. Edward Cowley. (Both men had been on the church committee that had investigated his case.) Cowley went to Albany with the petition and asked that a committee be appointed to investigate the Society, focusing on Edward Jenkins, the secretary and superintendent of the NYSPCC. The Senate said they would consider it, but later declined to investigate.

Cowley lived the remainder of his life quietly, out of the public eye, occasionally publishing papers of a religious nature. He died in his home at 223 E. Eighty-Eighth Street, on April 20, 1891, at age sixty-three. For the ten years after Cowley had been removed from the Children's Fold, eleven children died there.

When Cowley had traveled to Albany in a final attempt to clear his name, the Department of Public Charities and Correction paid $180,000 for Rikers Island (what the 413-acre island might cost today is incalculable). They would "build a magnificent penitentiary there," Commissioner Brennan told a senate committee, and everyone was all for the plan. "The shadow of the penitentiary rested upon all the noble works of charity upon Blackwell's Island," a *New York Times* article read. As long as institutions like the Penitentiary and the Almshouse remained together on the same tiny island, the popular viewpoint that there was little difference between the poor and the criminal was in danger of becoming entrenched forever.

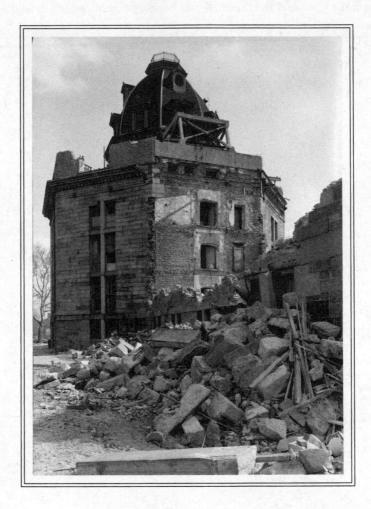

⊰ VI ⊱

SEPARATING CHARITY
FROM CORRECTION

---◆---

NEW YORK CITY DIVIDES THE
DEPARTMENT IN TWO IN 1895

THE END OF A DANGEROUS CONGLOMERATE

———◆———

I T IS NOT the order of God," Rev. French wrote, "that we should crowd the wretched of the world, least of all His loving children, into one great Lazar House." ("Lazar House" is another term for a leper colony.) One of the most destructive outcomes of this arrangement, French thought, was the now-fixed association between crime and poverty. "The dark shadow of crime spreads right and left, from the Penitentiary and the Workhouse, over all the institutions, the Asylum, the Alms-House and Charity Hospital; so that, in the minds of the people at large, all suffer alike from an evil repute." Being poor had become a character trait that needed "correction," like the impulse to steal or cheat. The Christian impulse to help the needy had been tamped down and replaced with an inclination to punish them.

French was one of many pointing out that Blackwell's Island had become a dangerous conglomerate. In 1886, Louis L. Seaman, the former chief of staff of Blackwell's Island hospitals, called the affiliation between crime and poverty a "diabolic Malaprop," insisting that "the relation between crime and poverty is no more essential than between crime and wealth." Where were the standing armies of police to monitor the crimes of the elite? Worse, the poor were not corrected on Blackwell's Island; they were destroyed. "No man or woman who is 'sent up' to these colonies ever returns to the city scot-free," Seaman railed. "There is a lien, visible or hidden, upon his or her present or future, which too often proves stronger than the best purposes and fairest opportunities of social rehabilitation."

The State Board of Charities was responsible for "every project or reform for betterment thus far attempted in our municipal institutions," Seaman wrote. While the commissioners of the Department of Public Charities and Correction, "together with its entire system from the greatest to the least, from centre to outpost, is in abject slavery to politics, is a recognized, hopeless appendage of the 'machine.' . . . The machine is supreme; and the commissioners rattle their own handcuffs of partisan servitude while reducing this array of employees and subordinates to the lock-step of partisan bondage."

Almost ten years later, in 1895, another group, the State Charities Aid Association, would finally push through what Seaman, French, and so many others saw as the most crucial step in unsnarling this vicious association: the separation of the Department of Public Charities and Correction into two distinct administrations, one overseeing charity and the other, correction. A bill to effect the division was sent to the Senate and the Assembly in Albany.

Most of the commissioners were opposed to the idea; one of their representatives, Louise Darche, the superintendent of the New York City Training School for Nurses, made their objection clear and demonstrated the reformer's point. "There is certainly no danger of moral contamination" to the City Hospital patients, she said. Because "at least 50 per cent of our patients are men and women who at some time or other been inmates of the almshouse, the workhouse, or the penitentiary." In other words, they were all the same. The Penitentiary and Workhouse wardens argued that rebuilding on Rikers the infrastructure they already had on Blackwell's would be an enormous and needless expense. The commissioners also saw the move as diluting their power. On February 1, 1895, there were 16,649 inmates and 1,903 officers and employees scattered among all the institutions under their control. That was the equivalent of 1.2 percent of the entire population of New York City at the time (equivalent to 98,000 people today), and all under the management of three men.

Despite their opposition, the bill passed both houses of the legislature. It only required approval from Mayor William Strong and a signature from Governor Levi Morton. To help Strong make a decision, a group from the State Charities Aid Association met in his office on May 7, 1895. Although Josephine Shaw Lowell had resigned from the State Board of Charities in 1890, she was asked to speak. She didn't hold back. She'd had contact with the Department of Public Charities and Correction for nineteen years, she reminded them, and continued her testimony: "I think I may safely say that I do not know of a single measure of radical reform which has emanated from a Commissioner of the department. By radical reform I mean anything which showed that the causes of crime and pauperism had even been studied. . . . The only apparent object has been to receive everybody sent into the institutions, to keep them in the cheapest way, and let them die or go, as the case might be when the time came."

"Every one who has made any real study of the department, during the last twelve years at least," she continued, "has recommended that a change and division be made. . . . And what the bill before you provides for, is that unfortunate men, women and children, who through accident or disease, beyond their own control, are thrown upon the charity of the city, should be relieved from the stigma and contamination of association with criminals. . . . [The] unnatural combination of criminals, paupers, insane, sick adults, diseased children and babies under the care of the department" must end.

William Strong had been elected as a reformer, and he did his best to deliver, most famously by appointing Theodore Roosevelt police commissioner and charging him with cleaning up the corrupt police department. Strong also established the New York City Board of Education. When he addressed the Board of Aldermen at the beginning of 1895 he said, "I am clearly of the opinion that the care of the indigent should be separate from the discipline of those who have broken the law. To continue these branches together prevents proper assistance to those incapable of self-support and prohibits the best results from being obtained from corrective discipline." Therefore it was no surprise when he turned to the assembled group and said he would "take great pleasure in approving this bill." They'd been waiting for this for years. The room erupted into applause and everyone jumped up to shake the mayor's hand. Progress could finally begin.

On June 5, 1895, Chapter 912, separating charities from correction, was signed into law by Governor Morton. Effective January 1, 1896, one department would become two: the Department of Public Charities and the Department of Correction.

French would not live to see the day the bill finally became law. "I have crossed the river, leaving out vacations and Saturdays, 9,056 times," he wrote in 1888, and "I have walked, on an average three miles each day, making 13,584 miles." But his eighty-first birthday was coming up on June 10, and he was tired. He'd already been relieved of most of his duties the previous fall. While other priests were seeing to the various institutions on the Island, most of French's work was now confined to the Almshouse. It wasn't a small responsibility. Over 4,000 people were now being admitted to the Almshouse every year. The decision was also made to have French split the Sunday services in his beloved Chapel of the Good Shepherd with his assistant, Rev. Charles C. Proffitt. It must have been the hardest task to relinquish. When passing by the more grand cathedrals of the city, French would often proudly proclaim, "I think if Christ came to New York, He would select our chapel on the island in preference to these fine churches." But his voice had grown so faint he couldn't be heard beyond the front pews.

In the spring of 1895, while the State Charities Aid Association was lobbying to divide up the Department of Public Charities and Correction, French was working hard to prepare inmates of the Almshouse in what would become his very last confirmation class. It was a race against time, for both the students and French. The men and women in his class were the "poorest of the poor, the miserable, the deaf, blind, dumb, old, sick and dying." Six of his students had already ended up on a table in the morgue. Towards the end of May, French also started feeling unwell.

It didn't stop him from boarding a steamer to the Island on Sunday,

May 26. He was scheduled to present his class for confirmation at Trinity Church on June 9, the day before his birthday, and there was still much to be done. Rev. Proffitt was supposed to give the sermon at the Chapel of the Good Shepherd that Sunday morning, but French stopped him. "I want to preach this morning; I feel that I must do so." Of course Proffitt stepped aside for the old priest. "The end of all things is at hand," French began.

He was dead less than twenty-four hours later.

On Wednesday morning, the same people who'd listened to his last service, and many others, began filing past the open casket.

French occasionally allowed himself to feel proud of what he'd managed to accomplish on the Island, particularly his libraries. In what would be his final annual report, he wrote, "It was my privilege to establish libraries in the Charity Hospital, the Penitentiary, the Workhouse," and to enlarge the ones that already existed in the Lunatic Asylum and the Almshouse. For many of those institutionalized on the Island those books were the only relief from their dreadful, comfortless surroundings.

But French's greatest gift may have been, simply, himself. Unlike most priests, who primarily saw the members of their congregations once a week on Sundays, French was among the inmates of Blackwell's Island almost every day. He was the friend, family member, and spiritual guardian they either never truly had, or once had and lost. For decades he listened to the beaten, broken, and largely abandoned inhabitants as they voiced their regrets about what they'd missed in life, and confronted what every human must one day face. All day long that Wednesday, hundreds and hundreds of old men and women slowly walked past the casket on either side, sobbing, "We have lost our best friend."

French, however, went to his grave unsure if he was truly making a difference. Elsewhere in his last annual report, he wrote, "The harvest is great and increasing, and the laborers are few, and one can only do a portion of the sowing and leave others to reap, with vain regrets that so little has been accomplished, still hoping that there has been enough gathered in to entitle the reaper the comforting word of commendation for what has been done."

French would also not live to see one other very important development that the State Charities Aid Association finally managed to bring about, and it was a harvest that he had helped to sow. When Mayor Strong had addressed the Board of Aldermen in January 1895 and announced that the Department of Public Charities and Correction should be divided in two, he also said, "The care of the insane in this county should pass to the State." The need for this action had been apparent for some time, and the State Charities Aid Association had been pushing for the transfer for years.

French was so outspoken about the city's wretched care of the insane that a commissioner of the Department of Public Charities and Correction once thought he was in league with the State Charities Aid Association. The commissioner's fears had been prompted by French's comments in an 1879 newspaper article: "One proof of the spirit which prevails there is even seen in the printed declaration which our mission finds it necessary to make, to the effect that our representatives have nothing to do with the fare, treatment, discipline or bodily condition of the patients, but only with their spiritual instruction. I have always taken exception to this view. I hold that it may be our duty as Christian to look after the bodies as well as the souls under our charge." French had been one of the only workers on Blackwell's Island to tell the 1880 Senate Committee on Insanity the truth about what was going on inside the Lunatic Asylum.

Unfortunately, the committee's investigation did not lead to change, and French likely felt he was a failure. "I would fain hope, for the good of the inmates," French wrote in 1882, "that at no distant day the Asylum would cease to be a prison; that through a generous and enlightened public opinion some plan may be devised, the result of experience in our own and other lands, whereby the officials can secure a larger percentage of lunatics 'made whole.'"

It wasn't that the commissioners were unaware that the care for the insane on Blackwell's Island was abysmal, but they weren't about to relinquish all that political power voluntarily. Pressure for reform was growing, however, and they had to do something. With encouragement from

Josephine Shaw Lowell, in 1887 the Board of Estimate and Apportionment approved the commissioners' request for money to buy 1,000 acres covered with scrub pine and oak out in Central Islip to build what they would call the City Farm. Instead of being locked up indoors with their delusions and rats, on the proposed farm the city's insane would have a daily occupation out in the sun, in a still more pastoral setting, far from the city and everything in it that could cause them harm. French was not optimistic. "They cannot make the institution what it ought to be and what I know they wish it to be." It was long past time to give someone else a chance to do better.

Construction of facilities on the farm proceeded haltingly, and although the Department transferred 314 male patients there in 1889, there were still thousands of men and women left in asylums on Blackwell's, Hart, and Wards Islands, where conditions continued to deteriorate. "Some of the buildings used as dormitories for the insane on Harts Island [sic], are a disgrace to civilization," an 1890 grand jury found. "The water supply on this Island is obtained from cisterns and driven wells. When it is known that 75,000 bodies lie buried in close proximity to these cisterns, one can readily imagine what the character of the water must necessarily be."

That year, due largely to the efforts of Louisa Lee Schuyler, founder of the State Charities Aid Association, the New York legislature passed what came to be known as the State Care Act. It placed the care of the insane in New York into the hands of the State Commission in Lunacy. Soon after, roughly 16,000 patients, or one-tenth of all the insane people in America, were transferred into the custody of the state.

The women trapped on Blackwell's Island and all the other inmates in the asylums managed by the Department of Public Charities and Correction were not among the rescued. The counties of New York, Kings, and Monroe were initially exempt from the State Care Act because they already had extensive infrastructure in place to care for their insane patients, and the state did not have enough room to accommodate their inmates. The city could have transferred its insane over to the state at any time, along with the buildings, land, and equipment that were used to house and care for them. Monroe had quickly decided this was better for everyone and had transferred its insane patients to the state. But the city and the commissioners were still not ready to give up control. Their exemption did not free them from their obligation to pay their share of taxes for state care, however, and they would protest what they saw as an unfair financial burden.

The following year Blackwell's Island Asylum inmate Julia Doyle was found floating in the river. She was supposed to be on suicide watch, but someone had apparently looked away. One hundred sixty-four other women would die in the Asylum that year, and every year the numbers would grow. One hundred eighty-four died in 1892. In 1893 the number surged to 297, the highest to date, and still the numbers rose. When 340 women died in the Asylum in 1894, just under 20 percent of all the women housed there that year—and more than any previous year—responding to the crisis became nothing less than a matter of life and death.

There had been an opportunity to push New York City to join the other counties and transfer care of its insane to the state in 1892, when Mayor Hugh Grant asked the State Commission in Lunacy to form an advisory committee to look into the existing conditions in the asylums. Despite reporting that each patient's life in city care had become "one long hopeless misery," the commission did not recommend transferring the remaining insane to state care and instead focused on separating the Department of Public Charities and Correction.

The commission did have some suggestions about improving life in the asylums. They were impressed with what the department had built so far in Central Islip, which they called an "admirable insane establishment." They also thought Wards Island was redeemable. They concluded their report by recommending that the department concentrate all its efforts on these two locations. Purchase more land in Central Islip and enlarge the facilities there; buy the remaining part of Wards Island, which was still owned by the state, and expand the properties there as well; then move all the insane from Blackwell's and Hart Islands to Wards Island and Central Islip, and either convert the vacated facilities to hospitals or tear them down.

The commissioners made an effort to act on these suggestions but, as always, there were delays in completing the new buildings. On March 15, 1894, 1,221 women were transferred to buildings on Wards Island that were still unfinished. That left 533 women remaining on Blackwell's, in the notorious Retreat and two brick pavilions. Everyone was about to learn that this was yet another horrible misstep in a half-century march to infamy and dishonor.

On May 13, 1894, the *New York Herald* published an article titled "Horrors of Bedlam." Following in the footsteps of Nellie Bly, a reporter named Adele Porter Porre had gotten herself hired as a nurse in order to report on conditions at Wards Island, where most of the city's insane were now housed. The commissioners had likely been congratulating themselves on migrating such a large number of patients to the new facilities, but now everyone was talking about how Porre's article read just like Nellie Bly's from 1887. "They were stripped and then plunged into the tub one after another . . . irrespective of whether any of them had any skin diseases or not." One woman who was embarrassed to be seen naked and too slow getting out of her clothes was grabbed by the hair and dragged violently into the bath. Afterwards they were sent back to their rooms dripping, shivering, and humiliated.

The women had been merely shuffled from one hell to another.

Mayor Thomas Gilroy asked the State Commission in Lunacy to look into each charge of abuse outlined in the *Herald* article. Commissioners Dr. Carlos G. Macdonald, Godwin Brown, and Henry A. Reeve began their investigation on May 31, 1894, hearing witnesses at the Park Avenue Hotel.

Much of the information in Porre's article had come from Dr. Louise G. Rabinovitch, who'd been hired as a result of Nellie Bly's suggestion to the grand jury that the presence of female doctors would greatly improve matters in the all-female Asylum. Rabinovitch was brought in as an assistant physician under Emmet C. Dent, the medical superintendent. After witnessing the horrors there, Rabinovitch started secretly copying records for a book she planned to write about the abuses on Blackwell's Island. She shared her stories and records with Porre and left her position two weeks before the article came out.

Over the course of the State Commission investigation, Rabinovitch revealed atrocities like the practice of keeping the women quiet by injecting them with morphine, chloral, and hyoscyamine at such dangerous doses that at least one patient, Hannah Fitzgerald, had died. The doctor who performed Fitzgerald's autopsy, Dr. Lyman A. Cheney, had determined that the cause of death was chloral poisoning, but Dr. Dent overrode his finding and put cerebral hemorrhage on the death certificate. Rabinovitch also claimed that necessary operations were often not performed. Madeline Reil, for example, complained frequently about pains she'd been having, but the doctors told her that the pains were imaginary. When she died, an autopsy revealed gallstones and peritonitis. "Gynecological treatment," Dr. Rabinovitch declared, "was not given to patients in the asylum because Dr. Dent did not believe in it. He claimed the brain was not affected by the condition of the abdomen."

After Rabinovitch's testimony, the commissioners of the Department of Public Charities and Correction hired lawyers. Henry H. Porter, the president of the Department of Public Charities and Correction, accused Rabinovitch of gross neglect. "She admits having witnessed the so-called abuses which she describes, but she did not attempt to have them remedied."

On June 15, Arthur H. Mastin, the counsel representing the Asylum managers, spent six hours trying to break Rabinovitch's testimony. From 10 a.m. to 5 p.m. he questioned her, with only one hour adjournment for lunch. When she tried to talk about the condition of the patients and the fact that they were starving, Mastin interrupted her. "I don't want to hear anything about starvation," he said. It was more important to him to learn how she came to testify. She was there, she answered, because the counsel for the *New York Herald* had asked her to testify.

The *New York Herald* reported that the Asylum authorities were "afraid of the cool little woman doctor," and they may not have been exaggerating. At one point Rabinovitch objected so forcefully to Mastin's questions that he voluntarily backed down. Rabinovitch had been to asylums throughout Europe, she told the commission, and never had she seen anything to compare to the mismanagement and atrocities on Blackwell's Island. When asked why she didn't report these cases to the State Board of Charities, she said it was because Dr. Dent told her that complaining to them would be unmannerly. Likely, she feared for her job.

There had been several attempts by management to intimidate witnesses. When the charges first appeared in the *Herald* article, Dr. Dent asked at least one attendant, Margaret Harrison, to sign a paper saying the charges were untrue. She refused and was reprimanded. Harrison went on to tell the commission that she once saw rats carry off a loaf of bread. A supervisor named Michael O'Brien told them that they continued to bathe multiple patients in the same tub without changing the bathwater. When he saw the displeased looks on the Asylum officials' faces, he quickly qualified his statements. "We didn't often bathe more than three in the same water." The lawyer representing the asylum officials that day asked if he knew this practice was against the rules. Yes, he answered, but "there was always a doctor present." If the officials looked irritated before, they must have looked positively enraged now. This indicated the doctors knew about the custom and did nothing to stop them. The lawyer immediately started berating O'Brien until he took back his statement, saying that they only did it when the doctors' backs were turned.

O'Brien was right to be nervous. One attendant, Susie Sherman, confessed that many of them were afraid to testify truthfully because they'd lose their jobs. A week after this admission, one of the *Herald*'s lawyers received a letter affirming that Susie Sherman had, in fact, been discharged, and that another attendant, Rose Jennings, who had testified that the meat stew they were served looked "like a pig's dish," had been transferred. Dr. Dent denied that these actions had anything to do with the women's testimony, but he was lying.

Dr. Carlos F. Macdonald, who was heading up the investigation, had a relatively cordial relationship with Alexander E. Macdonald, the general superintendent overseeing all of New York County's asylums. Alexander did not try to pretend everything was just fine for the insane of New York City, and Carlos was more than willing to address all the problems in a way that would avoid embarrassment for Alexander and all concerned. But after Susie Sherman was fired, Carlos wrote Alexander. "I don't see how you can afford to make an enemy of me just at this time," he began in fury. He'd recently helped Alexander through some professional difficulty (he doesn't say what), and he continues, "I am sure I should not have interceded in your behalf if I had know that you were instrumental in causing a poor innocent widow, Miss Sherman, with a half-orphan child to support, to lose her position." (This is the same man who fired the nurse who begged to have a dying patient who'd been assaulted taken to the hospital, and not the doctor who had refused.)

Although the Department of Public Charities and Correction brought forth a few attendants who denied the charges of abuse, witness after witness corroborated Rabinovitch's claims. Nurse Frances C. McIntire told the commission that the dormitories were so infested with rats that one burn patient, who was "too demented and weak to call out" was forced to lie there unattended as the "rats crawled up and gnawed the bandages off her body." The case was reported to the doctors, she said, but as usual nothing was done. Dr. James R. Garrard testified about a special accident book that was kept by attendants to note patient injuries. Doctors used this book to decide who needed treatment, but since attendants were frequently the cause of the "accidents," they simply neglected to enter the ones they didn't want the doctors to know about. Garrard also told them that another reason the women didn't get proper gynecological treatment was because the doctors weren't given the instruments they needed to provide it. Further, they had to get Dr. White's, the asylum's visiting surgeon, permission before performing any surgery, and Dr. White had only set foot in the Asylum twice so far that year.

Various ex-attendants, who had no reason to fear retaliation, testified, as did former patients. Former attendant Mattie Skillen said the attendants regularly "choked patients, pulled their hair, twisted their wrists, and bent back their thumbs." Colonel A. H. Rogers, who said that he'd personally witnessed many acts of brutality while a patient, called Wards Island a "slaughterhouse of the mind." There were a lot of accounts of attendants punishing men by employing what was called a "health lift," or "Irish hypodermic." Three or four attendants would pick up the patient, lift him over their heads, then dash him to the ground as hard as they could.

Dr. Lyman A. Cheney's testimony was particularly incriminating. As the commissioners sat back in easy chairs at the head of the parlor of the Park Avenue Hotel, Dr. Cheney confirmed that Hannah Fitzgerald died of chloral poisoning, and that he'd found no evidence to support a determination of cerebral hemorrhage. According to the *New York Times*, Cheney's finding didn't match what was on the death certificate, he said, because "he did not wish to argue with Dr. Dent, who was inclined to be disagreeable." Cheney also talked about getting Wards Island ready for the women. Among the many things the commission was trying to determine was what happened to the $500,000 that had been appropriated for new buildings on Wards Island and at the Central Islip Farm. Cheney said he was given two carpenters and one painter to work on the new buildings, but shortly after getting there one of the carpenters and the painter were pulled from the asylum projects and sent to work on Alexander Macdonald's new house instead.

The commission paid a call to Wards Island, but the administration had known a visit was inevitable and they'd had plenty of time to prepare. They'd scrubbed the place down, disinfected, and laid traps for the rats. They also cleaned up the inmates and had been feeding them lemon, eggs, whiskey, and cow's milk instead of condensed milk for weeks. The visit was not enlightening.

A 5,700-page report was released by the State Commission in Lunacy on December 26, 1894. In general, they defended the medical officers and the general superintendent, concluding they were not responsible for the current state of affairs, and that the general superintendent himself had repeatedly pointed out all the problems. A lot of the statements from former workers were written off as the vindictive testimony of disgruntled dismissed employees, and they sided with the doctors against all accusers, even if the accuser was another doctor. The commission also inexplicably downplayed serious problems like the lack of medical instruments and gynecological care for the female patients.

The commission didn't entirely excuse the administrators. They believed that the drugs Hannah Fitzgerald was given contributed to her death, but they did not recommend any action be taken against the doctors, writing only that, "the commission is of the opinion that the exhibition of such heroic doses of powerful drugs is inadmissible, and should under no circumstances be permitted." They also confirmed Cheney's claim that the $500,000 worth of bonds that had been issued to build additional accommodations were used, in part, to build an "expensive residence" for the general superintendent, and what little work had been done was shoddy.

While the commission's report can be seen as exonerating the city and the Department of Public Charities and Correction from most of the more sensational claims printed in the *New York Herald*, it may have been because the commission decided to concentrate on fixing the problem, rather than assigning blame. There was no need to establish that the system was a failure. That it had "developed inherent difficulties and defects, which experience has shown to be ineradicable, even under the ablest management," was known by all. After so many decades of trying, it was no longer reasonable to expect that the city would ever be able to fix it. The only effective course of action left was to transfer the care of the insane to the state. "The principle of State care for the dependent insane represents the most intelligent and humane thought upon the subject at the present time, and it is hoped that the local authorities in the counties of New York and Kings, who are responsible for the matter, will not long hesitate in taking the necessary steps for the complete consummation of this policy by availing themselves of the opportunity extended to them in the State care act."

General Superintendent Alexander Macdonald did not deny the commission's findings. He dismissed Dr. Rabinovitch, however, and her book, "which she afterwards sought, unsuccessfully, to dispose of, in the guise of a 'Work of Fiction' to different publishers." It seems pretty shabby of him, since he knew that her claims were absolutely true. But Macdonald was not above a spiteful response (like firing Susie Sherman). While conceding that the result of the investigation would be good for the inmates of the asylums, and that the problems would be fixed once and for all, he thought it was worth noting that the investigation had created all this extra work for them and had interrupted their routines.

The commissioners of the Department of Public Charities and Correction were not at all happy about being portrayed in such a negative light and wrote to Macdonald to ask him if the condition in the asylums "justifies such wholesale denunciation." Did he point out the improved diet to the Lunacy Commission? And the upgraded beds and mattresses? Were the investigators told that the commissioners had done "all in their power to improve the condition of the Asylum and their inmates, and in no instance refused to grant any request made?"

Macdonald's return letter reads like a man doing his best to tell the truth while still trying to hold on to his job. In response to their desire to know if the Lunacy Commission had been told that they'd done "all in their power," Macdonald wrote bluntly, "No." But he added, "No question was asked or conversation had that would lead to such a statement." As to whether or not conditions at the asylums "justifies such wholesale denunciation," Macdonald danced around for a few paragraphs before saying, "I would not, myself, select the word 'disgraceful' to characterize the condition of the Asylums; that it is 'distressing' is, in my belief, true." In an impressive demonstration of political spin, Macdonald wrote that the state spent twice what they did per patient, so when "compared then with the inmates of the State Asylums, the City patients may be said to be 'poorly clothed, poorly fed.'"

After the report, two new bills were introduced to the legislature. Under the first act, the asylums at Central Islip and Wards Island would be reorganized as the Manhattan State Hospital. The insane who remained on Blackwell's and Hart Islands would be under the control of the state as well, staying where they were until accommodations could be provided for them in the Wards Island or Central Islip facilities. The second bill addressed the asylums of Brooklyn, which would be reorganized as the Long Island State Hospital. The Brooklyn bill was signed into law by Governor Levi Morton on May 11, 1895.

Manhattan took a little longer, due to two years of back taxes for the care of the insane owed by the city to the state. As a result, 516 women remained on Blackwell's Island in buildings whose capacity taken together was 354. The women also no longer had a bathhouse because that was given to the hospital that had taken over the former Asylum main building. Meanwhile, the Board of Estimate and Apportionment had not approved any money that year for building and improvements for Blackwell's and all the other asylums, because they now anticipated that the insane were going to be transferred to the care of the state.

On June 7, Dr. Carlos Macdonald and his fellow commissioners sent a long letter to Governor Levi Morton. Because the Board of Estimate and Apportionment was withholding funds for repairs that year, the state of the 6,700 patients in all their asylums could only be characterized as nothing "less than a burning disgrace. . . . In the name of our common humanity and on behalf of these thousands of wretched people, we implore your Excellency . . . to act on this bill. Sign it, and so hasten the solution which must inevitably come sooner or later. . . . Affix your name to one of the great progressive steps that will honorably distinguish your administration for all time." Their letter was printed in all the papers.

Henry H. Porter, the President of the Department of Public Charities and Correction, wrote to Mayor Strong, to insist that "the Insane of this City and County are better housed, fed, clothed and generally cared for than they have been for many years" and that waiting for the next year's appropriation "will entail no suffering upon the inmates." He saw no reason to transfer their care to the state and assured Mayor Strong that "nothing will be left undone, to contribute to the care and comfort of thousands of inmates in the different Institutions of this Department."

Porter would not survive the coming break-up of the Department.

In September the courts decided that New York City had to pay the back taxes it owed to the state. There was no longer any reason to hold up the bill. Still, Governor Morton didn't sign it into law until January 28, 1896, using a gold pen made just for the occasion by Tiffany & Company and sent to him by Louisa Lee Schuyler, of the State Charities Aid Association, who had been so instrumental in getting the State Care Act passed. On February 28, 1896, the New York City Asylum for the Insane became the Manhattan State Hospital for the Insane, and with that act, they believed, "the last vestige of the cruel poorhouse system of caring for them has been swept away." The state now cared for 19,058 people, at an annual expense of $4.5 million, and the state was given five years to build suitable accommodations on Wards Island and Central Islip for the patients remaining on Blackwell's and Hart Islands. Dr. Alexander Macdonald ran what would be called Manhattan State Hospital East (the men's asylum on Wards Island), Dr. Emmet Dent ran Manhattan State Hospital West (the women's asylum on Wards Island), and Dr. George A. Smith, who was a superintendent at the Hart Island Asylum, ran what would eventually be called Central Islip State Hospital.

The State Charities Aid Association was confident that everyone would now get "better food, better nursing, better clothing, better buildings," and "a larger measure of comfort" than ever before.

Perhaps some of the association members looked back with satisfaction on the December 18, 1879, meeting at Cooper Union sixteen years earlier, when asylum reformers resolved that the "seriously defective system of the care of the Insane . . . should be abandoned in this country wherever it exists, as it has been abandoned in other countries." With the fire of a good and noble purpose, they'd proudly declared "that this great State of New York, an Empire in itself, can do nothing else more grand and good. Digging canals, chartering railways, founding schools, endowing universities, neither of them is so great, so urgent, so Divine a work, as caring in the best way possible for these afflicted and helpless ones."

That same passion must have possessed them now, amplified with triumph. The Asylum inmates were safely in the care of the state; plans were in the works to replace the crumbling Penitentiary and Workhouse with "the most perfect prison in all the world" on Rikers Island; leaving the Almshouse and all the various hospitals in the now-dedicated care of the Department of Public Charities, and away from all the ill effects of their former proximity to the convicted and the insane.

It was true that terrible mistakes had been made. But reformers and municipal workers were as optimistic as their predecessors were all those years ago, when they first planned a city of the poor on Blackwell's Island. This time they were going to get it right.

EPILOGUE

Blackwell's Island after 1895

———————◆———————

THEY DIDN'T GET it right.

In many ways, 1896 was just like 1895. A proposal to establish an electric-lighting plant on Blackwell's Island was abandoned, leaving surgeons to continue operating in the meantime by kerosene lamp, and everyone else to carry on in a nineteenth-century shroud of darkness. The female lunatics were still housed in the Retreat, the convicts remained huddled in their stone-cold caves, and the Almshouse was without running water and so crowded a houseboat was built and docked at the Twenty-Sixth Street Pier to accommodate the overflow.

Although Public Charities and Correction were now two separate departments, and the people working in the remaining asylums were employed by the state, everyone still shared the same crumbling buildings on the same grim islands. Workhouse inmates assigned to work in other institutions on the islands traipsed about as freely as before, despite the separation act that prohibited using prison help in any wards after January 1896. The Workhouse was renamed the Correction Hospital in 1916, and by 1924 it had evolved into a combined workhouse/penitentiary for women only, although it retained a separate hospital section for men.

The act also banned adding any more prison facilities on Blackwell's

Island, but instead of beginning the migration to Rikers, a new wing was constructed on the north side of the Penitentiary in 1897, bringing the total of inhumanly small cells to 1,104. The prison facilities on Rikers Island would not be built and occupied until 1936, after Mayor Fiorello La Guardia ordered his new correction commissioner, Austin MacCormick, to conduct a secret raid on Blackwell's. The Penitentiary had grown so corrupt by this time that three gangs were essentially running the place. For MacCormick and his men it was like invading a foreign and hostile country. The excrement bucket brigade that had been established over one hundred years before continued right up until the last group of prisoners were transferred to Rikers. The Penitentiary was torn down in 1936, and the Workhouse, aka Correction Hospital, came down the year after that.

The city knew history was not going to look back kindly on what had transpired on Blackwell's Island, and it tried to preempt future criticism in a statement buried in the cornerstone of the new penitentiary on Rikers, and published in the newspapers the day after the cornerstone-laying ceremony. They hoped that the recrimination to come would be "tempered by the thought that we did the best we knew how in the light of such knowledge and understanding as was given us." This new penitentiary, however—which they once thought they could build "for $200,000 or $250,000 with our own labor," but ultimately cost the city $10 million—was going to be, according to the commissioner speaking at the ceremony, "an institution designed to return the prisoner to society better than when he entered it, not worse, as is the case today."

Rikers is now recognized as one of the worst prisons in the United States. Life inside is so savage inmates call it "Rikers Island Gladiator School." After only three years it was already so crowded, unsanitary, and dangerous a Bronx court declared it "nearly unlivable." The 1941 Department of Correction annual report also noted the rise in "negro commitments." The percentage of men in the new workhouse on Rikers who were black went from 14 to 30 percent, and in the penitentiary from 17 to 32 percent. Black women, who were already incarcerated at higher rates than black men, rose to the majority among women. Their percentage increased from 32 to 58 percent in the workhouse, and from 41 to 54 percent in the penitentiary.

The most unpardonable offense, which continues today, is the practice of charging children sixteen years and older as adults and then throwing them in prison with men who are all too willing to rape and brutalize them—acts of abuse that are not committed by their fellow prisoners alone. Kalief Browder was arrested in 2010 at age sixteen for stealing a backpack and then held for three years without a trial on Rikers Island. During his time on Rikers, Kalief was beaten by both guards and inmates, and he spent an inconceivable two years in solitary confinement before his case was finally dismissed in 2013.

The next year the U.S. Justice Department published the results of a two-year investigation of Rikers that had uncovered a "deep-seated culture of violence" towards teenagers. Teachers and other staff members, it was learned, were instructed by correction officers to look away during assaults more horrific than anything Charles Dickens could imagine. One inmate was dragged from a classroom by a group of officers who then threw him to the ground and immediately began kicking and beating him while another teacher pulled her students away from the windows. When another officer came by and asked if he could join in, the others answered, "Sure, why not." Still another officer came by and "asked if anyone had pepper sprayed him yet, and then proceeded to spray him directly in the eye, one inch from his eye." The teacher later said she could hear the boy screaming and crying for his mother. On more than one occasion, inmates needed metal plates implanted in their skulls after unprovoked attacks by guards.

At the end of 2014, the U.S. Justice Department joined a class-action suit which had already been brought by the Legal Aid Society and others in 2011 (*Nunez v. City of New York*). Negotiations between the city and the Justice Department commenced. On June 6, 2015, Kalief Browder, who never recovered from the trauma of his incarceration, hanged himself from his bedroom window in the Bronx. The city settled on June 22. Sixteen- and seventeen-year-old inmates, the mayor announced, would no longer be placed in solitary confinement. At the time, New York and North Carolina were the only states in the country that still incarcerated adolescents with adults.

A new law passed in 2017, to take effect in October 2018, raises the age of criminal responsibility in New York to eighteen. It is not clear where the newly designated offenders will be jailed, but it won't be on Rikers. All sixteen- and seventeen-year-olds are to be removed by 2018. Rikers itself may be phased out. In 2017, Mayor Bill de Blasio announced that he supported a plan to close Rikers in ten years.

In 1896 New York State was given until 1901 to move all the inmates in the Lunatic Asylums to the facilities on either Wards Island or Central Islip. The state made its deadline, but because it wasn't able to build accommodations quickly enough, the women were transferred to a building that was neither safe nor sanitary. The East and West hospitals on Wards Island were consolidated and, after Alexander Macdonald resigned in 1904, Emmet Dent, a villain in Nelly Bly's report, became the superintendent of what was called the "largest psychopathic hospital in the world." The consolidated institution still operates and is now called the Manhattan Psychiatric Center. The Central Islip State Hospital, which became the Central Islip Psychiatric Center, closed in 1996. The growing trend of deinstitutionalization and the emergence of psychotropic medications led to a wave of asylum closings, which left many former patients on the streets.

City Hospital relocated to Elmhurst, Queens, in 1957 and was renamed Elmhurst General Hospital (now called NYC Health + Hospitals/Elmhurst). After that only two hospitals remained on Blackwell's: Welfare Hospital for Chronic Disease, which opened on the southern end of the Island in 1939 and was later renamed Goldwater Memorial Hospital, and Bird S. Coler Hospital, which opened on the northern end in 1952. Goldwater Memorial Hospital was originally a beautiful and humanely designed hospital, with windows positioned to allow sunlight to flood the rooms and corridors throughout the day. But budget cuts and cheap alterations made it so bleak and depressing that it was used as a location for the movie *The Exorcist*, when filmmakers wanted to show a character tormented with guilt for leaving his aging and ailing mother in a hospital for the poor. Goldwater and Coler were combined in 1996 and renamed NYC Health + Hospitals/Coler in 2015. City Hospital was demolished in 1994, and Goldwater Memorial Hospital, built on the site of the former Penitentiary, was torn down in 2015, to make room for the new Cornell Tech campus.

The name of the Almshouse was changed several times. In 1934, when it was called the New York Home for Dependents, the Depression had driven patient numbers so high that they were occupying abandoned Asylum pavilions. In its final incarnation it was called the New York City Home. It closed in 1953 after transferring all ambulatory inmates to a facility on Staten Island called the Farm Colony. Those requiring medical care were sent to the Bird S. Coler Hospital. The Farm Colony closed in 1975.

The Department of Public Charities was renamed the Department of Public Welfare in 1920, and Blackwell's Island was renamed Welfare Island in 1921. This was at a time when the word *welfare* did not elicit contempt, and looking out for the less fortunate members of society was considered a noble calling. The Department of Public Welfare became the Human Resources Administration in 1966, and today it is called the New York City Human Resources Administration/Department of Social Services.

By the 1950s Blackwell's Island was largely abandoned; it was re-envisioned in the 1960s as a progressive community of racially diverse and mixed-income residents, where everything would be handicapped-accessible. Residential development began in 1969, and the name of the island was changed again, in 1973, to Franklin D. Roosevelt Island, although it is always referred to simply as Roosevelt Island.

Building after building came down to make way for new construction, until almost all the nineteenth-century structures were gone. The only older buildings remaining today are the Lighthouse, built in 1872 on the northern tip of the Island, James Renwick's Smallpox Hospital, which went up in 1856, the Strecker Memorial Laboratory, a research facility that opened in 1892, and the octagon section of the Lunatic Asylum, which was restored and is now part of an exclusive apartment complex. (A residential home built between 1796 and 1804 for James Blackwell, a member of the family that once owned the island, still stands as well.)

Over a hundred years have passed since municipal leaders thought they'd identified all the problems in the system and put us on a path to fixing them. Adequate healthcare for the poor is currently in jeopardy, and the homeless and the mentally ill are back on the streets, except when we imprison them in jails that are in some ways worse than they were in the nineteenth century. Penitentiary Warden Joseph Keen's lament in 1851 about "the power of money to evade the law and escape its penalty" continues to be true today. To this day, people with money who commit crimes are not hunted and incarcerated to the degree that poor people are. As they have since the beginning, they pay their fine—if one is even imposed—and remain free.

The connection between crime and poverty persists, as does the idea that helping the poor only teaches dependency. In 1994, then-representative Newt Gingrich would say that welfare programs "ruin the poor. They create a culture of poverty and a culture of violence which is destructive of this civilization," as if tax breaks and what are called "incentive programs" when applied to the wealthy ruin them, or that their crimes are fewer and less destructive.

Josephine Shaw Lowell once strongly believed as Gingrich and others do. "Common charity," she wrote to her sister-in-law in 1883, "that is, feeding and clothing people, I am beginning to look upon as wicked! Not in its intention, of course, but in its carelessness and its results, which certainly are to destroy people's character and make them poorer and poorer." People meant well, she acknowledged, but their efforts only made matters worse. The poor "must be changed." She wrote a couple of years later, "They must be taught to love what is good, noble, and beautiful; they must learn self-respect, self-reliance, independence, before their condition can be changed."

But after decades of visiting the poor, and studying the institutions and programs meant to address issues of poverty, in 1894 she came to the conclusion that charity had not caused that predicament. The "want in which they now find themselves is not due usually to moral or intellectual defects on their own part, but to economic causes over which they have had no control and which were as much beyond their power to avert as if they had been natural calamities of fire, flood or storm."

"If the charity organization societies of the country are going to take the position of defenders of the rich against the poor, which I do think is the danger that stands before us," she warned later that year, "then I shall be very sorry that I ever had anything to do with the work."

The first step in getting it right is correctly identifying what is truly wrong.

ACKNOWLEDGMENTS

I COULDN'T HAVE WRITTEN this book without the help of my editor, Amy Gash; my agent, Amy Hughes; and my friend Howard Mittelmark. No one ever sees a thing I write until Howard has edited it first.

In my research I am indebted to Kenneth Cobb, the Assistant Commissioner at the NYC Department of Records and Information Services; Nathalie Belkins, Archivist at the NYC Department of Records and Information Services; Wayne Kempton, Archivist Historiographer Registrar at the Episcopal Diocese of New York; Judith Berdy, President of the Roosevelt Island Historical Society; Sister Monica Plante, Archivist for the Sisters of Charity of the Immaculate Conception; Sarah Currie, the Executive Director of the Williamstown Historical Museum; Joseph T. Gleason, Archivist at the New York Society of the Prevention of Cruelty to Children; Thomas McCarthy, Webmaster for the New York Correction History Society; Joseph van Nostrand, Archivist at the Division of Old Records, County Clerk of New York County; Arlene Shaner, Historical Collections Librarian, the New York Academy of Medicine Library; and Thomas Lannon, Acting Charles J. Liebman Curator of Manuscripts, the New York Public Library.

APPENDIX

THE HISTORY OF THE NAMES OF THE DEPARTMENT
OF PUBLIC CHARITIES AND CORRECTION

1734–1832	The Commissioners of the Alms House, Bridewell and Penitentiary
1832–1860	The Alms House Department
1860–1895	The Department of Public Charities and Correction
1895–1920	The Department of Public Charities
1895–Today	The Department of Correction of the City of New York
1920–1938	The Department of Public Welfare
1938–1970	The Department of Welfare
Today	The New York City Human Resources Administration/Department of Social Services (HRA/DSS)

THE INSTITUTIONS OF THE DEPARTMENT OF PUBLIC CHARITIES
AND CORRECTION IN 1893, PRIOR TO SEPARATION

BLACKWELL'S ISLAND

Almshouse
Asylum for the Indigent Blind
City Hospital
Hospital for Incurables
New York City Asylum for the Insane (formerly the Lunatic Asylum)
New York City Training School for Nurses
Penitentiary
Workhouse

(As of 1875 the Smallpox Hospital was controlled by the Board of Health, and later renamed Riverside Hospital. Riverside Hospital was moved to North Brother Island in 1885, and the former Smallpox Hospital was used as a home for the nurses from the Training School.)

HART ISLAND

City Cemetery
New York City Asylum for the Insane

LONG ISLAND

New York City Asylum for the Insane, Central Islip

MANHATTAN

Bellevue Hospital
Bureau of Medical and Surgical Relief for the Poor
City Prison (the Tombs)
Colored Home and Hospital
District Prisons (Five prisons in five districts)
Fordham Hospital
General Drug Department
Gouverneur Hospital
Harlem Hospital
Mills Training School (to train male nurses)
Morgue
Out-door Poor Department

RANDALL'S ISLAND

Infants' Hospital
Randall's Island Hospital and Schools

WARDS ISLAND

New York City Asylum for the Insane
Wards Island Hospital

SOURCE NOTES

A complete list of sources would increase the page count of this book by a third or more. Therefore I'm confining my source notes to a list of major sources, and within each chapter section, a selection of additional sources unique to that chapter.

ARCHIVES

Municipal Archives

Almshouse Ledger Collection, 1758–1953.

Board of Health Minutes.

City Cemetery, 1881–1950s.

Coroner and Office of Chief Medical Examiner, 1823–1950.

Court of General Sessions (felony cases), 1684–1920.

Mayors' files, 1849–present.

New York County District Attorney, 1895–1971.

New York County Court of General Sessions Grand Jury Indictments, 1879–1893.

Police Court/Magistrate's Court docket books, 1799–1930.

Municipal Library

Hard copies of the annual reports of the Governors of the Alms House, the Alms House Commissioner, and the Commissioners of Public Charities and Correction of the City of New York.

The Roosevelt Island Historical Society

The Blackwell's Almanac.

The New-York Historical Society

Patricia D. Klingenstein Library

Foote, J. D. *A Historical Account of the Persecutions and Imprisonments of J. D. Foote, in the New York Penitentiary, and State's Prison at Sing Sing.* 1810[?].

From pulpit to prison, from prison to pulpit: vindication of the Rev. Edward Cowley.
Robert Stewart Buchanan papers. 1825–1873 (bulk ca. 1845–1873), box that says "Sing Sing"
   (Adelaide Irving letters).
The Church and the Rev. Edward Cowley: a letter to the clergy of the Protestant Episcopal Church
   in the Diocese of New York. 1882.
Report of the Special Committee on the Establishment of a Workhouse, and the reorganization of
   the Alms House Department, 1842.
Addresses delivered on laying the corner stone of the intended penitentiary, on the island in the
   East River (late Blackwell's): in the presence of the mayor and the Common Council of the city of
   New-York, September 10, 1828, John, Stanford 1754–1834.

**The George Sim Johnston Archives of the New York Society
for the Prevention of Cruelty to Children**
New York Society for the Prevention of Cruelty to Children Annual Reports, 1881, 1882, 1885,
   1886, 1892.
Items from a folder titled "Willam H. Ramscar."

County Clerk of New York, Division of Old Records
Supreme Court (1799–1910).
Superior Court of the City of New York (1828–1895).

The New York Public Library
Alexander Jackson Davis papers, 1791–1937.
Maps Division and Local History Division, Blackwell's/Welfare/Roosevelt Island Maps, 1782–1885.
New York (State). Committee appointed to investigate the several department of the government
   of the city and county of New York. Investigation on the departments, vol. 2, 1885, pp. 1760–1797,
   testimony of Thomas S. Brennan.
Women's Prison Association of New York records, 1845–1983.

The New York Academy of Medicine, Archives and Manuscripts
Records of City Hospital (Welfare Island, N.Y.), 1877–1961, New York Academy of Medicine
   Library. (The name of Blackwell's Island was changed to Welfare Island in 1921.)
Alexander E. Macdonald Papers and Photographs, 1865–1906.

Oskar Diethelm Library
DeWitt Wallace Institute for the History of Psychiatry, Weill Cornell Medical College.

ANNUAL REPORTS AND MINUTES
Annual Reports of the Alms House Commissioner.
Annual Reports of the Board of City Magistrates of the City of New York.
Annual Reports of the Commissioner of the Alms House Department.
Annual Reports of the Commissioners of Public Charities and Correction of the City of New York.
   (No annual reports were issued for 1872, 1873, 1874, 1894, 1895.)
Annual Reports of the Governors of the Alms House, New York.
Annual Reports of the New York City Department of Correction.
Annual Reports of the New York Protestant Episcopal City Mission Society.
Annual Reports of the New York Society for the Prevention of Cruelty to Children.

Annual Reports of the Police Department of the City of New York.

Annual Reports of the Police Justices of the City of New York.

Annual Reports of the State Charities Aid Association.

Documents of the Senate of the State of New York, vol. 7. Transcripts of the 1880 Lunacy
Investigation.

Minutes of Committee of Direction, New York Protestant Episcopal City Mission Society.

Minutes. Meeting of the Commissioners of Public Charities and Correction.

Proceedings of the Board of Aldermen.

Proceedings of the Board of Assistant Aldermen.

Proceedings of the National Conference of Charities and Correction.

Report of the Commissioners of the Almshouse, Bridewell and Penitentiary.

DIARY

History of the Order of the Holy Cross at Valle Crucis North Carolina under Right Rev. Levi
Silliman Ives 1847–1851, written by Rev. William Glenney French, First Superior of the Order and
edited by his eldest son, H. Glenney French. Southern Historical Collection, University of North
Carolina. [French's diary.]

BOOKS, THESES, DISSERTATIONS

Berdy, Judith, and the Roosevelt Island Historical Society. *Roosevelt Island.* Mount Pleasant, S.C.:
Arcadia Publishing, 2003.

Burrows, Edwin G., and Mike Wallace. *Gotham: A History of New York City to 1898.* New York:
Oxford University Press, 2000.

Cray, Robert E. *Paupers and Poor Relief in New York City and Its Rural Environs, 1700–1830.*
Philadelphia: Temple University Press, 1988.

Dearborn, Frederick M. *The Metropolitan Hospital: A Chronicle of 62 Years.* [privately printed], 1937.

Friedman, Lawrence M. *Crime and Punishment in American History.* New York: Basic Books, 1993.

Gilfoyle, Timothy J. *City of Eros: New York City, Prostitution and the Commercialization of Sex,
1790–1920.* New York: W.W. Norton, 1992.

Gilfoyle, Timothy J. *A Pickpocket's Tale: The Underworld of Nineteenth-Century New York.*
New York: W.W. Norton, 2006.

Klips, Stephen Anthony. "Institutionalizing the Poor: The New York City Almshouse 1825–1860."
PhD diss., City University of New York, 1980.

Richmond, John Francis. *New York and Its Institutions, 1609–1871.* New York: E. B. Treat, 1871.

Scull, Andrew. *Social Order/Mental Disorder: Anglo-American Psychiatry in Historical Perspective.*
Berkeley: University of California Press, 1989.

Stewart, William Rhinelander, ed. *The Philanthropic Work of Josephine Shaw Lowell; containing
a biographical sketch of her life, together with a selection of her public papers and private letters.*
New York: Macmillan, 1911.

Waide, Susan P. "The Heritage of Roosevelt Island: A Content Analysis of Materials Present in the
Roosevelt Island Branch of the New York Public Library and Other New York City libraries and
repositories." M.L.S. thesis, Queens College, City University of New York, 1999.

Waugh, Joan. *The Unsentimental Reformer: The Life of Josephine Shaw Lowell.* Cambridge, Mass.:
Harvard University Press, 1998.

ONLINE SOURCES

The Social Welfare History Project.
http://socialwelfare.library.vcu.edu/organizations/care-insane-new-york-1736-1912/
HathiTrust's Digital Library.
https://www.hathitrust.org/
Ancestry.com.
www.ancestry.com
New York, Governor's Registers of Commitments to Prisons, 1842–1908.
http://search.ancestry.com/search/db.aspx?dbid=8870 (They have records for Blackwell's from
1883–1906.)
New York Correction History Society, produced by Thomas C. McCarthy.
http://www.correctionhistory.org/

PROLOGUE

Adams, William E. *Our American Cousins: Being Personal Impressions of the People and Institutions
of the United States*. London: Walter Scott, 1883.
Collins, Ace. *Stories Behind the Great Traditions of Christmas*. Grand Rapids, Mich.: Zondervan,
2003.

"Horses Shocked. Report That They Were Disturbed by Electricity Doubted." *New York Times*,
August 25, 1882.
"Edison's Electric Light. 'The Times' Building Illuminated by Electricity." *New York Times*,
September 5, 1882.

I: THE NEW YORK CITY LUNATIC ASYLUM. OPENED ON BLACKWELL'S ISLAND 1839, TO ACCOMMODATE NEW YORK CITY'S LUNATIC POOR.

Reverend William Glenney French: The Blackwell's Island Episcopal Missionary from 1872 to 1895

Assembly of the State of New York. *Report of the committee appointed by the Assembly of the
Legislature of 1830, to investigate the manner in which the Hospital in the city of New-York, and
the Asylum connected therewith, have disbursed the funds received by them*. Documents of the
Assembly of the State of New York, Fifty-Fourth Session, 1831, Vol. 3.
Board of Assistants. "To the Asylum Committee of the Board of Assistants from James
Macdonald." Document No. 48, Documents of the Board of Assistants. May 21, 1832–May 12,
1834. Vols. 2 and 3.
Boardman, Samantha. *The New York City Lunatic Asylum on Blackwell's Island: Madness and
Mayhem in Manhattan during the 19th century*. Institute for the History of Psychiatry Annual
Report to the Friends, July 1, 2004–June 30, 2005. Interdisciplinary Research Faculty, Richardson
History of Psychiatry Research Seminar, Oskar Diethelm Library.
Dickens, Charles. *American Notes*. New York: Penguin, 2000.
Gamwell, Lynn, and Nancy Tomes. *Madness in America: Cultural and Medical Perceptions of
Mental Illness Before 1914*. Ithaca: Cornell University Press, 1995.

Nicholls, Charles Wilbur de Lyon. *The Decadents: A Story of Blackwell's Island and Newport.* New York: J.S. Ogilvie, 1899.

National Institute of Mental Health. *Anxiety Disorder Among Adults.* https://www.nimh.nih.gov/health/statistics/prevalence/any-anxiety-disorder-among-adults.shtml

Ordronaux, John. *Commentaries on the Lunacy Laws of New York: And on the Judicial Aspects of Insanity at Common Law and in Equity, Including Procedure, As Expounded in England and the United States.* [Albany]: J. D. Parsons, Jr., 1878.

"Proceedings of the Third Meeting of the Association of Medical Superintendents of American Institutions for the Insane, Resolutions Respecting the Receptacle for Pauper-lunatics at Blackwell's Island." *New-York Journal of Medicine and the Collateral Sciences* 1, 1848.

Phillips, Wendell C. "The Bright and Dark Side of Hospital Life." *Alumni Journal,* April 1896. Published by the Alumni Association of the College of Pharmacy of the City of New York.

"Blackwell's Island Lunatic Asylum." *Harper's New Monthly Magazine,* February, 1866.

"Shocking Murder by a Lunatic on Blackwell's Island." *New York Times,* February 15, 1869.

"Horrible Affair at the Blackwell [sic] Island Insane Asylum." *New York Times,* February 16, 1869.

"The Lunatic Asylum Homicide—Action of the Coroner." *New York Times,* February 16, 1869.

"Treasures from Cyprus—New Statuary." *New York Times,* December 8, 1872.

"A Once-Grand Tower Is Given a New Life." *New York Times,* January 23, 2005.

Sister Mary Stanislaus: Committed to the Lunatic Asylum on Blackwell's Island, August 3, 1872, Diagnosis: Monomania

Sister Mary Stanislaus Is Admitted into the Asylum

The Trial of Sister Mary

The three chapters concerning Sister Mary were informed by correspondence with Sister Monica Plante, Sisters of Charity of the Immaculate Conception (SCIC) Archivist; Sister Timothea Kingston, a Holy Cross Sister and Assistant Archivist; items from the archives of the Sisters of Charity of the Immaculate Conception, Saint John, N.B. (listed below); and other sources listed below.

Annual Reports of the state of the New York Hospital and Bloomingdale Asylum, 1863–1892.

Assembly of the State of New York. Charges of the Bar Association of New York Against George G. Barnard and Albert Cardozo and John H. McCunn: And Testimony Thereunder Taken Before the Judiciary Committee of the Assembly of the State of New York, 1872, Vol. 3.

Chambers, Julius. *News Hunting on Three Continents.* New York: Mitchell Kennerley, 1921.

Coroners Office of the Borough of Brooklyn. Certificate and Record of Death for Rose McCabe (Sister M. Stanislaus) No. 2335, issued February 6, 1900.

Earle, Pliny. "History, Description, and Statistics of the Bloomingdale Asylum for the Insane, State of New York, America." *Journal of Psychological Medicine and Mental Pathology,* April 1, 1849.

Entry for Rose McCabe from the Medical Register of Bloomingdale Asylum, 1866–1890, No. 24.

Hennessey, M. Genevieve. *Honoria Conway: Woman of Promise, Foundress of Sisters of Charity of the Immaculate Conception, Saint John, N.B.* S.C.I.C.: 1985.

"Honoria Conway." *Dictionary of Canadian Biography.* http://www.biographi.ca/en/bio/conway_honoria_12E.html

Kennedy, Sister Estella. "Immigrants, Cholera and the Saint John Sisters of Charity: The first ten years of the Sisters of Charity of the Immaculate Conception, Saint John, N.B. 1854–1864." S.C.I.C. http://www.cchahistory.ca/journal/CCHA1977/Kennedy.html

Letter from Bishop Thomas Louis Connolly to Bishop James Rogers, December 28, 1861, S.C.I.C Archives.

Letter from Bishop James Rogers to Bishop John Sweeney, February 8, 1862, S.C.I.C Archives.

Letter from Seminarian John O'Leary to Bishop James Rogers, March 27, 1862, S.C.I.C Archives.

Letter from Bishop John Sweeney to Bishop James Rogers, March 30, 1862, S.C.I.C Archives.

Letter from Seminarian John O'Leary to Bishop James Rogers, March 31, 1862, S.C.I.C Archives.

New York State Senate. *Lunacy Investigation, A Special Committee of the New York State Senate.* Documents of the Senate of the State of New York, 105th Session, 1882, Vol. 7.

Ordronaux, John. "Letter to the Editor of the Albany Law Journal." *Albany Law Journal,* January 3, 1877.

Warrant of Commitment from Police Justice John McQuade, August 3, 1872.

Writ of Habeas Corpus in Supreme Court for Rose McCabe, aka Sister Mary Stanislaus, August 3, 1872.

"Lunatic Asylum Mystery." *Cincinnati Commercial,* August 8, 1872.

"Treatment of the Insane." *The Sun,* August 8, 1872.

"The Lunatic Nun." *Boston Globe,* August 15, 1872.

"The Bloomingdale Lunatic Asylum." *Evening Post,* September 3, 1872.

"Sister Mary of Stanislaus." *New York Herald,* September 4, 1872.

"The M'Cabe Lunacy Case." September 4, 1872, *New York Times.*

"The Case of Rose McCabe." *Commercial Advertiser,* September 5, 1872.

"Sister Mary of Stanislaus." *New York Herald,* September 5, 1872.

"Sister Mary of Stanislaus." *New York Herald,* September 6, 1872.

"End of the Lunacy Case." *New-York Tribune,* September 6, 1872.

"The McCabe Lunacy Case." *New York Times,* October 9, 1872.

"The Rose M'Cabe Insanity Case." *New York Herald,* November 2, 1872.

"The McCabe Lunacy Case." *New York Times,* November 2, 1872.

"The Doctors on Rose McCabe." *The World,* November 2, 1872.

"The Rose M'Cabe Case Again." *New York Herald,* November 3, 1872.

"The McCabe Lunacy Case—Further Testimony on the Part of the Defense." *New York Times,* November 10, 1872.

"The McCabe Lunacy Case." *New-York Tribune,* November 18, 1872.

"Rose M'Cabe Again." *New York Herald,* November 22, 1872.

"Sister Mary Stanislaus. Latest Movements and Future Intentions of the Persecuted Nun." *New York Times,* January 4, 1874.

"Sister of Charity Fatally Burned." *New York Herald,* February 4, 1900.

"Sister of Charity Burned." *New York Times,* February 4, 1900.

Suicide, Murder, and Accidental Deaths on the Rise in the Lunatic Asylum

Eckert, William G. "Medicolegal investigation in New York City: History and Activities 1918–1978." *American Journal of Forensic Medicine and Pathology* 4, no. 1 (1983).

New York State Senate. *Lunacy Investigation, A Special Committee of the New York State Senate.* Documents of the Senate of the State of New York, 105th Session, 1882, Vol. 7.

Ordronaux, John to Hon. William Laimbeer, President of the Board of Commissioners of Charities and Correction, May 23, 1874, Documents of the Senate of the State of New York, Ninety-Eighth Session, 1875.

Public Charities of New York City. An Appended Paper from the Thirteenth Annual Report of the Board of Charities of the State of New York, Made to the Legislature, February 5, 1880.

"A Dead Child." *New York Daily Tribune*, December 20, 1876.

"Encouraging Professional Beggars." *New-York Tribune*, December 23, 1876.

"That Mother's Dead Child." *New-York Daily Tribune*, January 2, 1877.

"Poisoned by Mistake." *New-York Tribune*, May 7, 1878.

"A Novelty in Mixed Drinks." *New York Times*, May 7, 1878.

"Fixing the Responsibility." *New York Herald*, May 10, 1878.

"Crime or Negligence." *New York Herald*, March 28, 1879.

"Emily Graham's Death." *New York Times*, March 28, 1879.

"Mrs. Graham Not Ill-Treated." *New York Times*, March 29, 1879.

"Treatment of the Insane." *New York Times*, November 1, 1879.

"Tormenting the Insane." *New York Times*, November 7, 1879.

"Treatment of the Insane." *New York Times*, November 14, 1879.

"Blackwell's Island Abuses." *New York Herald*, November 16, 1879.

"Insane Asylum Abuses." *New York Times*, November 19, 1879.

"An Insane Woman Killed." *New York Times*, January 29, 1880.

"The Lunatic Homicide." *New York Times*, January 30, 1880.

"Maria Ottner's [*sic*] Death." *New York Herald*, February 4, 1880.

"Medical Treatment of the Insane." *New-York Daily Tribune*, February 6, 1880.

"The Ottmer Inquest." *New York Times*, March 16, 1880.

"Burned to Death." *New York Times*, April 5, 1880.

Lunacy Investigation, December, 1880, Metropolitan Hotel, New York City

New York State Senate. *Lunacy Investigation, A Special Committee of the New York State Senate.* Documents of the Senate of the State of New York, 105th Session, 1882, Vol. 7.

Nellie Bly, *Ten Days in a Mad-House*, September, 1887

Bly, Nellie. "Among the Mad." *Godey's Lady's Book*, January 1, 1889.

———. *Ten Days in a Mad-House*. New York: Ian L. Munro, 1887.

Chambers, Julius. *News Hunting on Three Continents*. New York: Mitchell Kennerley, 1921.

Dent, Emmet C. "Hydriatic Procedures as an Adjunct in the Treatment on Insanity." *American Journal of Psychiatry* 59, no. 1 (July 1902).

"Grateful to Mr. Wagener." *New York Times*, November 1, 1887.

"Thinks She Was Abused." *New York Times*, March 2, 1888.

"Charging Her Death to the Nurses." *New-York Tribune*, March 2, 1888.

"Insane and Diseased." *New York Times*, March 3, 1888.

II: THE WORKHOUSE. A PENAL INSTITUTION FOR PEOPLE CONVICTED OF MINOR CRIMES, OPENED ON BLACKWELL'S ISLAND IN 1852.

New York City and the Unworthy Poor

Charity Organization Society of the City of New York. Committee on Criminal Courts. *The Forgotten Army: Six Years' Work of the Committee on Criminal Courts of the Charity Organization Society of the City of New York, 1911-1917*. New York: Committee on Criminal Courts of the Charity Organization Society of the City of New York, 1918.

Cobb, W. Bruce. *Inferior Criminal Courts Act of the City of New York*. New York: Macmillan, 1925.

Faber, Eli. *The Trial Transcripts of the County of New York, 1883–1927*. New York: John Jay Press, 1989.

"The Farce of Police Court Justice in New York: Magistrates, Lawyers, Ward Heelers, Professional Bondsmen, Clerks of the Court and Probation Officers join to Make a Mockery of 'The Supreme Court of the Poor.'" *Broadway Magazine* 17, no. 5 (February 1907).

Freedman, Estelle B. *Their Sister's Keepers: Women's Prison Reform in America, 1830-1930*. Ann Arbor: University of Michigan Press, 1984.

Harris, Mary B. *I Knew Them in Prison*. New York: Viking Press, 1942.

Paddon, Mary E. "Inferior Criminal Courts of New York City." *Journal of Criminal Law and Criminology* 11, no. 1, 1920.

Police Court—Second District, Magistrates Court Docket Books, Roll #4.

"John Doe." *New York Herald*, March 14, 1875.

"The Case of Jacob B. Stockvis." *New York Times*, March 24, 1875.

Rev. William R. Stocking, Superintendent of the Blackwell's Island Workhouse from 1886 to 1889

Annual Report of the State Board of Charities for the Year 1887, The Work-House, New York City, Report to the State Board of Charities by Josephine Shaw Lowell, July 12, 1887.

Annual Report of the Women's Prison Association, 1888.

Bly, Nellie. "Why Don't Women Reform." *New York World*, June 17, 1888.

Lowell, C. R. "One Means of Preventing Pauperism." Paper presented at the Sixth Annual Conference of Charities, Chicago, June 1879.

Board of Charities of the State of New York. "Public Charities of New York City." An Appended Paper from the Thirteenth Annual Report of the Board of Charities of the State of New York, made to the Legislature, February 5, 1880.

Stocking, W[illiam] R[edfield] "The City Workhouses and Their Problems." *New Outlook* 41 (1890).

Stocking, William Redfield. *The Story of My Life*. Williamstown, Mass.: Williamstown Historical Museum.

Stocking, W[illiam] R[edfield] to Hon. Abram S. Hewitt, January 30, 1888, Mayor's files, Municipal Archives.

"The Work-House—Blackwell's Island." *W. H. Harper's New Monthly Magazine*, June 1, 1866.

"Blackwell's Island Abuses, Letter to the Editor by Miss Morgan." *New York Herald*, November 24, 1879.

"An Extraordinary Story." *New York Times*, March 21, 1880.

"Mrs. Little and Her Nephew." *New York Times*, May 28, 1880.

"Convicted of Perjury." *New York Times*, May 30, 1880.

A Workhouse Exposé and Lawrence Dunphy, Superintendent of the Blackwell's Island Workhouse from 1889 to 1896

Rogers, William P. "A Month in the Workhouse." *New York World*, June 10, 1888.

Stocking, William Redfield. *The Story of My Life*. Williamstown, Mass.: Williamstown Historical Museum.

Stocking, William R[edfield] to Hon. Thomas S. Brennan, President of the Department of Public Charities and Correction, June 18, 1888, Mayor's files, Municipal Archives.

III: THE ALMSHOUSE. COMPLETED IN 1848, TO HOUSE THE POOR AND DISABLED OF NEW YORK CITY.

The Almshouse Complex, The End of the Line for Many

Annual reports of the Colored Home, 1861–1877.

Annual Reports of the Association for the Benefit of Colored Orphans, 1861.

Barnes, T.H. *My Experiences as an Inmate of the Colored Orphan Asylum New York City*. Written in 1924, copyright Fanny Crawford, Douglass Barnes Crawford, Miriam I. Wexner Crawford, 2005.

Brown, Junius Henry. *The Great Metropolis, a Mirror of New York*. Hartford, Conn.: American Publishing Company, 1869.

Cook, Adrian. *The Armies of the Streets: The New York City Draft Riots of 1863*. Lexington: University Press of Kentucky, 2014.

Folks, Homer. "Reform and Public Charities." *Outlook*, March 6, 1897.

Harris, Leslie M. *In the Shadow of Slavery: African Americans in New York City, 1626–1863*. Chicago: University of Chicago Press, 2004.

Hulkower, Raphael. "From Sacrilege to Privilege: The Tale of Body Procurement for Anatomical Dissection in the United States." *Einstein Journal of Biology and Medicine* 27, no. 1 (2011).

New York City Board of Aldermen. The Alms House Proper, Report of the Commissioners of the Alms House, Penitentiary and Bridewell, September 11, 1837, Documents of the Board of Aldermen of the City of New York, From No. 1 to No. 90, Inclusive—May 1837–May 1838, Vol. 4.

New York City Common Council. Minutes, 1784–1831, vol. 9, April 20, 1818.

New York City County Coroner Inquests, Roll 90, Municipal Archives.

New York City Department of Health. "Investigation of methods of transportation of corpses and foodstuffs on boat 'correction.'" Department of Health, Sanitary Bureau, April 8, 1918, Mayor's files, Municipal Archives.

New York City Department of Public Charities. A statement of facts, New York, City Club of New York, 1903.

New York City Office of the Coroner, February 10, 1863 to August 8, 1863, Roll 4023, Municipal Archives.

New York County District Attorney Indictment Records, Roll 120, Box 769, Municipal Archives.

New York State Assembly. No, 31, in Assembly, January 25, 1854, Remonstrance of the Irish Emigrant Society, against the bill "To promote medical science." Documents of the Assembly of the State of New York, Seventy-Seventh Session, 1854, vol. 1.

New York State Legislature. Laws of the State of New York passed at the session of the Legislature, 1854. Chap. 123, An Act to promote Medical Science, p. 282.

SenGupta, Gunja. *From Slavery to Poverty: The Racial Origins of Welfare in New York, 1840–1918.* New York: NYU Press, 2009.

Seraile, William. *Angels of Mercy: White Women and the History of New York's Colored Orphan Asylum.* New York: Fordham University Press, 2011.

Thompson, Mary W. *Sketches of the History, Character, and Dying Testimony, of Beneficiaries of the Colored Home, in the City of New-York.* New York: J. F. Trow, 1851.

"The Turpin Legacy." *Colored American,* December 30, 1837.

"Fiendish Murder of a Negro: The Perpetrator in Custody—He Is Positively Identified." *New York Times,* August 1, 1863.

"In the Potter's Field." *New York Times,* March 3, 1878.

"Current Topics (discusses Act of 1879)." *Albany Law Journal,* May 28, 1891.

"More Victims of Typhus." *New York Times,* January 5, 1893.

"Blackwell's Island Abuses; Overcrowded, Poor Food, and Inadequate Hospital Facilities, Letter to the Editor by Dr. William G. Le Boutillier." *New York Times,* February 11, 1894.

"Its Sixtieth Anniversary: Founding of Colored Home and Hospital Celebrated." *Baltimore African-American,* May 13, 1899.

"Hospital Work in New York." *Baltimore African-American,* December 23, 1911.

"Colored Asylum is 100 Years Old." *New York Times,* December 6, 1936.

IV: THE HOSPITALS FOR THE POOR. IN OPERATION BEGINNING 1832, TO SERVE THE SICK PEOPLE OF NEW YORK CITY, AND THE INMATES OF THE PENITENTIARY, WORKHOUSE, AND ALMSHOUSE.

Penitentiary Hospital aka Island Hospital aka Charity Hospital aka City Hospital

Garrigues, Henry Jacques. *Practical Guide in Antiseptic Midwifery: In Hospital and Private Practice,* [Detroit]: George S. Davis, 1886.

"Leading the Way: Our Island and the March of Medicine Part 1—City Hospital." *Blackwell's Almanac: A Publication of the Roosevelt Island Historical Society* 1, no. 3.

Lister, Joseph. The Antiseptic Method of Dressing Open Wounds. A Clinical Lecture. Delivered at Charity Hospital, New York, October 10, 1876, Medical Record, vol. 11.

New York (State). Committee appointed to investigate the several department of the government of the city and county of New York. Investigation on the departments, vol. 2, 1885, pp. 1760–1797, testimony of Thomas S. Brennan.

Phelps, Abel M. "Transplantation of tissue from lower animals to man, and a report of the case of bone-transplantation at Charity Hospital, Blackwell's Island, N.Y." *Clinical Orthopaedics and Related Research* 371 (February 2000). (Includes a brief modern commentary on the experiment.)

Sanger, William. *The History of Prostitution: Its Extent, Causes, and Effects throughout the World.* New York: Harper, 1858.

Society of the Alumni of City (Charity) Hospital. Report for 1904, together with a history of the City Hospital and a register of its medical officers from 1864 to 1904 / committee on Publication, Charles G. Child, Jr., Walter C. Klotz, J.W. Draper Maury.

Testimony Taken Before the Senate Committee on Cities Pursuant to Resolution Adopted January 20, 1890, Vol. 4, Henry H. Porter 1885 testimony, p. 3367.

"The Training of a Nurse." *Scribner's Magazine* 8, no. 5 (November 1890).

U.S. Federal Census. 1880 Schedules of Defective, Dependent, and Delinquent Classes, Page 3, Enumeration District No. 556, June 1, 1880, Epileptic and Paralytic Asylum, Blackwell's Island.

"Blackwell's Island Hospitals." *New York Times*, May 24, 1855.

"The Board of Governors." *New York Times*, May 30, 1855.

"Blackwell's Island Hospital Destroyed by Fire." *New York Herald*, February 14, 1858.

"Alleged Murder at Blackwell's Island." *New York Times*, May 3, 1867.

"The Blackwell's Island Outrage." *New York Times*, May 7, 1867.

"Conclusion of the Examination in the Blackwell's Island Case." *New York Times*, May 12, 1867.

"A New Disinfectant." *Chicago Daily Tribune*, July 1, 1876.

"A New Thing in Surgery. Transfusion of Human Milk into the Veins of Charity Hospital Patient—Not a Successful Operation." *Louisville Courier Journal*, April 15, 1879.

"The Charity Hospital." *New York Times*, July 28, 1883.

"No Cure for Consumption Yet: The New Remedy Declared a Failure." *New-York Tribune*, September 11, 1887.

"A Novel Surgical Operation." *New York Times*, November 19, 1890.

"Both Boy and Dog are Doing Well." *New York Herald*, November 19, 1890.

"Dr. Phelps' Experiment." *New York Times*, November 26, 1890.

"The Boy and the Dog." *New York Times*, December 9, 1890.

"Johnny Gethius and His Bone Graft." *New York Herald*, December 14, 1890.

"The Boy and the Dog." *New York Times*, February 7, 1891.

"Practically a Success: Bone Grafting as a Science Fully Explained." *Boston Daily Globe*, February 20, 1891.

"Bone Grafting Not a Success." *New York Herald*, February 20, 1891.

"The Boy and the Dog." *New-York Tribune*, February 20, 1891.

"Report on Recent Bone Grafting." *The Sun*, February 20, 1891.

"Grafting a Dog's Bone to a Boy." *Chicago Daily Tribune*, February 22, 1891.

"Poor Little Johnny." *Elmira Daily Gazette and Free Press*, May 16, 1891.

"Aquzon in Phthsis: Ozone Preparation Used with Good Effect, It Is Claimed." *Chicago Daily Tribune*, February 6, 1893.

"Martyr to Surgical Hypnotism." *Cincinnati Enquirer*, May 20, 1894.

"Charcotism Proves to Be a Fake." *Cincinnati Enquirer*, September 6, 1896.

"Streetscapes/Charity Hospital on Roosevelt Island; Piles of Rubble Where Grim Gray Walls Once Stood." *New York Times*, October 16, 1994.

V: THE PENITENTIARY. COMPLETED IN 1832, FOR PEOPLE CONVICTED OF MORE SERIOUS CRIMES, AND WITH SENTENCES GENERALLY LONGER THAN SIX MONTHS.

Adelaide Irving, Sentenced to the Penitentiary, December 6, 1862

Child, L. Maria. *Letters from New-York*. New York: Charles S. Francis, 1842.

Letter from Adelaide Irving to Mrs. E. C. Buchanan, undated, but likely around July, 1866.

Letter from Adelaide Irving to Mrs. E. C. Buchanan, October 12, 1866.

McCabe, James D., Jr. *The Secrets of the Great City: A Work Descriptive of the Virtues and the Vices, the Mysteries, Miseries and Crimes of New York City*. Philadelphia: Jones Brothers, 1868.

McCarthy, Thomas C. "Penitentiary Origins in the City of New York." New York Correction History Society.

"Court of General Sessions: An Interesting Case—Does a Non-Companionable Husband Own His Wife's Money." *New York Times*, October 25, 1862.

"Court of General Sessions—October 24—Before Recorder Hoffman." *New-York Tribune*, October 25, 1862.

"Romantic History of a Young Female Criminal." *Albany Evening Journal*, August 10, 1865.

"The Case of Adelaide Irving." *New York Herald*, August 10, 1865.

"A Letter from the City Prison." *New York Herald*, August 15, 1865.

"A Female There Trapped." *New York Herald*, May 10, 1869.

"A Female There Doing a Wholesale Business." *New York Times*, May 10, 1869.

"A Sad Case—A Young Lady Becomes an Habitual Thief." *New York Times*, May 25, 1869.

"Sing Sing's Prison's Dead." *The Sun*, July 20, 1879.

"The Blackwell's Island Homicide." *New York Herald*, June 10, 1879.

"Doing Time on the River." *The New York Times*, February 9, 2012.

William H. Ramscar, The Old Gentlemen's Unsectarian Home, Sentenced to the Penitentiary, December 23, 1889

Letter from Elbridge T. Gerry to the Board of Health of the City of New York, March 26, 1886.

Letter from Wm. H. Ramscar to E. T. Gerry, April 19, 1886.

New York City County Coroner. Evidence on Inquisition held on Bessie Slocum, June 1882. Filed June 7, 1882, Municipal Archives, New York City County Coroner, Roll 96.

Report of the Foundling Asylum of the Sister of Charity in the City of New York, January 1 1882– January 1 1883.

"Doubtful Conduct of a Policeman." *New-York Tribune*, March 30, 1882.

"Large Death Rate in an Asylum." *New York Times*, May 24, 1882.

"Mr. Ramscar's Sanatorium." *New York Herald*, May 25, 1882.

"Bessie Slocum's Death." *New York Times*, June 3, 1882.

"Where Little Ones Die." *New York Times*, June 6, 1882.

"Ramscar's Case in Court." *New York Times*, June 8, 1882.

"The Case of Ramscar." *New York Times*, June 10, 1882.

"The Case of Ramscar." *New York Times*, June 16, 1882.

"Mr. Ramscar Set at Liberty." *New-York Tribune*, June 17, 1882.

"City and Suburban New." *New York Times*, June 17, 1882.

"The Unsectarian Home Closed." *New-York Tribune*, June 18, 1882.

"Red Tape Protecting Criminals: The Coroners Not at All Pleased with the Decision in The Ramscar Case." *New York Times*, June 20, 1882.

"Ramscar's Old Men's Home." *New-York Tribune*, April 4, 1886.

"Ramscar Bobs Up Again." *New York Times*, May 6, 1886.

"Ramscar in Court Again." *The World*, February 11, 1888.

"Beat an Old Man." *New York Times*, August 13, 1889.

"Ramscar Again Brought to Justice." *New-York Tribune*, August 13, 1889.

"Ramscar Is at It Again." *The World*, September 16, 1889.

"Ramscar Found Guilty." *New York Times*, December 19, 1889.

"Ramscar Sentenced." *New York Times*, December 24, 1889.

"Ramscar to the Front Again." *New York Times*, August 14, 1892.

"Preys on Misery." *New York Herald*, November 24, 1895.

"Ramscar Carried off to Jail." *The Sun*, March 13, 1910.

Reverend Edward Cowley, The Shepherd's Fold, Sentenced to the Penitentiary, February 20, 1880

Annual Report of the Shepherd's Fold of the Protestant Episcopal Church in the State of New York, 1870, 1871.

Children's Fold. Annual Reports for 1878, 1881, 1882, 1886.

Cowley, Edward. *From Pulpit to Prison, from Prison to Pulpit: Vindication of the Rev. Edward Cowley*. [Self-published,] 1881.

K., Rajakumar. "Vitamin D, Cod-liver Oil, Sunlight, and Rickets: A Historical Perspective." *Pediatrics* 112, no. 2 (August 2003).

Louis Victor: His Sickness and His Cure. [Self-published,] 1885. https://archive.org/details /louisvictorhissioounse

New York State Board of Charities. Extract from the Ninth Annual Report of the State Board of Charities of the State of New York Relating to Orphan Asylums and other Institutions for the Care of Children, 1876.

Ogden, David B. *The Church and the Rev. Edward Cowley: A Letter to the Clergy of the Protestant Episcopal Church in the Diocese of New York*. [Self-published,] 1882.

An Open Letter to Elbridge T. Gerry Esq. from Rev. Edward Cowley, June 1, 1882.

Report of the committee of investigation, in the case of Rev. Edward Cowley. June 6, 1881, New York: A. Livingston, 1881.

"Brutal Treatment of Children." *New York Times*, January 15, 1877.

"Charges Against a Charity." *New-York Tribune*, January 15, 1877.

"The Children's Fold." *New York-Tribune*, January 16, 1877.

"Cruelty at the Children's Fold." *New York Herald*, January 17, 1877.

"The Shepherd's Fold." *New York Herald*, March 15, 1878.

"Charity Disgraced." *New York Herald*, January 18, 1880.

"The Shepherd's Fold Case." *New York Times*, January 19, 1880.

"The Shepherd's Fold." *New York Herald*, January 20, 1880.

"Tender Mr. Cowley." *New York Herald*, January 25, 1880.

"A Shepherd and His Fold." *New York Times*, January 25, 1880.

"Shepherd Cowley's Fold." *New York Times*, January 29, 1880.

"How the Children Were Starved." *New York Times*, February 1, 1880.

"Shepherd Cowley's Defense." *New York Times*, February 12, 1880.

"The Shepherd's Fold." *New-York Tribune*, February 12, 1880.

"Mr. Cowley's Trial Closed." *New York Times*, February 17, 1880.

"Cowley in the Penitentiary." *Chicago Tribune*, March 3, 1880.

"Where He Belongs." *St. Louis Dispatch*, March 4, 1880.

"The Shepherd's Fold." *New York Times*, June 4, 1880.

"Shepherd Cowley Free." *New York Times*, January 15, 1881.

"Shepherd Cowley's Case." *New York Times*, July 23, 1881.

"'Shepherd's Fold' Cowley." *New York Herald*, July 23, 1881.

"My Year in Stripes." *The World*, August 18, 1894.

VI: SEPARATING CHARITY FROM CORRECTION.
NEW YORK CITY DIVIDES THE DEPARTMENT IN TWO, 1895

The End of a Dangerous Conglomerate

Department of Correction. Special Centennial Issue, June, 1995, Chapter 912 Split Public Charities and Correction.

Department of Public Charities of the City of New York Statement of Facts, published by the City Club of New York, May, 1903.

Fifty-First Annual Report of the Prison Association of New York, 1895.

Greater New York Charter, submitted to the Legislature of New York on February 20, 1897, by the Commission appointed pursuant to Chapter 488 of the Laws of 1896, Chapter XIX, New York Charter, Department of Correction.

Investigation of the departments of the City of New York. v.2, by New York (State). Legislature. Senate. Special Committee to Investigate the Departments of the City of New York. Published 1885.

Letter from the Commissioners of the Department of Public Charities and Correction to Governor Levi P. Morton, June 17, 1895. (Municipal archives, Mayor's files.)

Letter from Henry H. Porter to Mayor William Strong, July 18, 1895. (Municipal Archives, Mayor's files.)

Letter from Carlos F. MacDonald to Alexander E. Macdonald, August 16, 1894. (Macdonald Papers.)

Letter from George F. Britton, Secretary, Department of Public Charities and Correction, to Alexander E. Macdonald, June 13, 1895. (Macdonald Papers.)

Letter from Alexander E. Macdonald to Henry H. Porter, President, Department of Public Charities and Correction, June 20, 1895. (Macdonald Papers.)

Report of the Grand Jury of New York for the January Term of 1890, the Court of General Session of the Peace, of the City and County of New York [concerning visits to the institutions under the care of the Department of Public Charities and Correction].

Report of the proceedings for establishing a Board of Commissioners in Lunacy, for the State of New York. Supervision of our Asylums for the Insane, A. G. Sherwood, 1880.

Seaman, Louis L. "The Social Waste of the City." *Science* 8, no. 190 (September 24, 1886).

State Charities Aid Association of New York. Report on the Department of Public Charities of New York City, from the Twenty-Fourth Annual Report of the State Charities Aid Association to the State Board of Charities, October 1, 1896.

Third Annual Report of the State Charities Aid Association to the State Commission in Lunacy, December 1, 1895.

Twenty-Third Annual Report of the State Charities Aid Association, December 1, 1895.

"Outrages on Lunatics." *Evening Telegram of New York*, October 31, 1879.

"Protestant Episcopal Missions." *New York Times*, October 31, 1879.

"Insane Men as Farmers." *New York Times*, February 14, 1892.

"Horrors of Bedlam." *New York Herald*, May 13, 1894.

"To Investigate Asylums for the Insane." *New York Times*, May 18, 1894.

"Patients in Living Tombs." *New York Times*, June 8, 1894.

"Doctors Left Them To Die." *New York Times*, June 9, 1894.

"Dr. Rabinovitch's Charges Denied." *New York Times*, June 10, 1894.

"Rats Gnawed the Bandages." *New York Times*, June 15, 1894.

"Enough to Make Reason Totter." *New York Herald*, June 15, 1894.

"Not Matched for Barbarity." *New York Times*, June 16, 1894.

"Proof from Records Now." *New York Herald*, June 21, 1894.

"Would Shield Her Informers." *New York Times*, June 21, 1894.

"Abuse of the Insane." *New York Times*, June 22, 1894.

"A Mental Slaughterhouse." *New York Times*, June 23, 1894.

"Did Not Produce His Books." *New York Times*, June 27, 1894.

"Told by a Doctor." *New York Herald*, June 29, 1894.

"Investigators at Wards Island." *New York Times*, June 29, 1894.

"Food for Insane Patients." *New York Times*, July 21, 1894.

"Hardships of the Insane." *New York Times*, July 27, 1894.

"Careless of Patient's Health." *New York Times*, July 28, 1894.

"State and City Care of the Insane." *New York Times*, December 18, 1894.

"Opposed to Pavey Bill; A Mistake to Divide the Department of Charities and Correction." *New York Times*, March 15, 1895.

"Mayor Strong Will Sign." *New York Times*, May 8, 1895.

"The Prisoner's Paster: An Apostolic Life on Blackwell's Island." *The Churchman*, June 15, 1895.

"The Appointments Made." *New York Times*, December 22, 1895.

"To Separate 'Charities and Correction.'" *New York Times*, December 26, 1895.

"Lunacy Board's Powers." *New York Times*, May 15, 1896.

Epilogue: Blackwell's Island after 1895

Dworkin, Hildy. *Selected History and Evolution of The Human Resources Administration*.

Fifty-First Annual report of the Prison Association of New York for the Year 1895.

First Annual Report of the Manhattan State Hospitals, to the Board of Managers, for the year ending September 30, 1905.

Geismar, Joan H. An Archaeological Evaluation of the Northtown Phase II Project Area, Roosevelt Island New York, prepared for the Starrett Housing Development Corporation. April 26, 1985.

Giraudet, Charles. *Autopsy of a Hospital: A Photographic Record of Coler-Goldwater on Roosevelt Island.* Urban Omnibus, 2014.

Grand Jury investigation into Penitentiary for Males and Correctional Hospital for Females on Welfare Island, October 15, 1924.

Lowell, Josephine Shaw. "Methods of Relief for the Unemployed." *The Forum*, February 1894.

New-York Historical Society. *A History of City Home, produced by the Department of Hospitals, from a collection of printed material pertaining to the New York City Home for Dependents Indentures, 1718-1727, 1792-1915.*

Report of the Welfare Island Planning and Development Committee: submitted to John V. Lindsay, Mayor, City of New York, February 1969.

Second Annual Report of the Managers of the Manhattan State Hospital at New York, to the State Commission in Lunacy, for the year ending September 30, 1897.

Sixth Annual Report of the Managers of the Manhattan State Hospitals at New York, to the State Commission in Lunacy, for the year ending September 30, 1901.

Stuhler, Linda S. *The Inmates of Willard 1870 to 1900, Manhattan State Hospital, Ward's Island, New York City.*

U.S. Department of Justice, United States Attorney Southern District of New York Report, CRIPA Investigation of the New York City Department of Correction Jails on Rikers Island, August 4, 2014.

"To Build a Bigger Jail." *New York Times*, September 20, 1886.

"A Barge for Homeless Men." *New York Times*, March 10, 1896.

"New Almshouse Buildings." *New York Times*, October 29, 1897.

"Blackwell's Island, A Prison Terrible." *New York Times*, March 27, 1914.

"Mayor Lays Stone for Penitentiary." *New York Times*, July 29, 1931.

"Prison Builders Deny City Charges." *New York Times*, January 20, 1934.

"Welfare Island Little More Than a Name to New Yorkers." *New York Times*, February 11, 1934.

"City Prison Shut after 110 Years." *New York Times*, February 8, 1936.

"Folk at City Home Fear Moving Day." *New York Times*, August 24, 1952.

"Aged Completing City Home Exodus." *New York Times*, May 13, 1953.

"Welfare Is. May Be Roosevelt Is., Metropolitan Briefs." *New York Times*, January 21, 1973.

PHOTOGRAPH AND MAP CREDITS

New York Public Library Map

https://digitalcollections.nypl.org/items/510d47e2-09a8-a3d9-e040-e00a18064a99

The Library of Congress Image of the Lunatic Asylum Octagon before Demolition:

Library of Congress, Prints and Photographs Division, HABS, Reproduction number HABS NY,31-WELFI,6--2. Photographer, Jack Boucher.

Museum of the City of New York Images:

Penitentiary:
Jacob A. (Jacob August) Riis (1849–1914) / Museum of the City of New York. 90.13.1.13.

Almshouse:
Jacob A. (Jacob August) Riis (1849-1914) / Museum of the City of New York. 90.13.1.89.

Workhouse:
Jacob A. (Jacob August) Riis (1849-1914) / Museum of the City of New York. 90.13.1.12.

New York Academy of Medicine City Hospital Image:

Image of City Hospital from the Alexander E. Macdonald Papers and Photographs Collection, Courtesy of The New York Academy of Medicine Library.

Municipal Archives Image of Octagon:

Asylum dpc_1606, Collection name: DPC: Public Charities and Hospitals, Courtesy NYC Municipal Archives.

INDEX

RESURRECTING FORGOTTEN LIVES:
THE MILLIONS INTERVIEWS STACY HORN
by Sarah Cords

———————◆———————

STACY HORN DEFIES death by ceaselessly writing books about it. Her new book is a history of New York City's Blackwell's Island (renamed Roosevelt Island in 1971), the site of several nineteenth-century institutions in which death was no stranger but rather a frequent visitor. In *Damnation Island*, Horn resurrects the stories of many who have been forgotten, including the missionary who walked a route between all the island's facilities (including the Lunatic Asylum, the Workhouse, the Almshouse, the Penitentiary, and several hospitals) and talked with their inmates daily; the "lunatic nun" who fought to get herself released from the asylum; and a young girl who received her first prison sentence at fifteen.

Recently I got to have what turned out to be a surprisingly cheerful email conversation with Horn about death, resurrection, community, and, oh yes, fact-checking.

The Millions: Stacy, I loved your new book. But it's full of unhappy stories that mostly end unhappily. Can you tell me what drew you to Blackwell's Island? What made you think, "I want to investigate this history of the 'poor, sick, mad, and criminal' and spend years writing about it"?

Stacy Horn: I desperately wanted to find happy endings. I'm always drawn to sad stories, but sad stories that are mostly forgotten, precisely because I hope that by resurrecting these people and what happened, I will bring a sense of peace to their histories, and to the reader.

Blackwell's Island drew me in because I already had a general sense of what had gone on there. I knew I would have thousands and thousands of opportunities to recover what was forgotten, and to use their stories to enlighten the present.

What I didn't get was happy endings. Instead, I'm now a passionate advocate for criminal justice and mental health care and welfare reform.

The Millions: In the book, you follow several personal stories, including those of the Reverend French, who was a missionary to Blackwell's Island, and multiple inmates and staff members of the various institutions there. How did you find those stories, and how did you decide on the people whose stories you told in detail?

Stacy Horn: It's a good thing that research, and the chase, is my favorite part of writing, because this book was my biggest challenge to date. Not surprisingly, most of the records for each of the institutions on Blackwell's Island (the Lunatic Asylum, the prisons, the Almshouse, etc.) were not saved.

I was able to tell the stories I did through a combination of luck and perseverance. For example, at the New-York Historical Society, I came across a letter from a young woman imprisoned in Sing Sing to a society lady who had visited her once. Something about that letter drew me to the inmate, Adelaide Irving, whom I ended up featuring in the Penitentiary section of my book. But there were no official Penitentiary records of Adelaide because none were saved. I had to kind of reverse-engineer her story from a number of other sources, and here I was lucky that any existed at all.

Sister Mary, the "lunatic nun" who was committed to the asylum, was an even bigger challenge because there are still fewer extant records for the asylum. Here again I lucked out because I happened to find an archivist nun in Canada who was willing to help me, and the Sisters of Charity of the Immaculate Conception turned out to be better recordkeepers than the city of New York. Reverend French wrote annual reports, thank God, and a wonderful Workhouse warden wrote an autobiography, as did a survivor of the attack on the Colored Orphan Asylum during the draft riots in 1863. All these little miracles helped me to recreate what life was like on Blackwell's Island during the nineteenth century.

Oh, and remembering researching Adelaide Irving just reminded me of a very proud find I made. After being told that there were no prison records for the Penitentiary at all anywhere, from every librarian, archivist, and corrections history expert I consulted, I found the records for 1883 to 1908 on, of all places, Ancestry.com. I was searching on a generic Irish name, because most of the inmates were Irish, and a number of Blackwell's Island Penitentiary inmates popped up. I'm sure I screamed. The actual records are at the State Library in Albany, where I'd already looked, but they were indexed in such a way that no one knew they were there. I went back and let everyone who'd told me that they didn't exist know, but they weren't as excited as me. No one screamed. Come on! Nineteenth-century prison records, people!

The Millions: I am blown away by the scope and sources of this book. How long did it take to research it? Was there a point when you knew you had to stop researching, and start writing?

Stacy Horn: I never stop researching. When I start writing that only leads to more research. Even when a book is finished and published, I will still keep looking into whatever subject I've written about. I still research cold cases and unsolved murders after writing about the NYPD's Cold Case Squad, and I keep up with parapsychological research after writing about the former Parapsychology Laboratory of Duke University.

I never let go. I must have attachment issues. But I started researching Blackwell's towards the end of 2014. I started writing in probably around the summer of 2015, and I was still working on it this year, right up until the moment my editor insisted I "step away from the computer, Stacy."

The Millions: I want to talk about how that theme of never letting go appears in your other work, and talk about your other books, but I also want to ask about something as workaday as fact-checking. I know you are very dedicated to doing that for all of your nonfiction. Do you literally go through your manuscripts line for line and make sure everything has a source, a citation? How long must that have taken for this one?

Stacy Horn: With every book I get better and better at fact-checking. I've learned over time that yes, you really do have to check almost every line. It's insane how, no matter how careful you are, mistakes creep in. It also takes such a ridiculously long time that knowing how much work I have ahead of me I'm always a little nauseous before I begin. I may even cry a little. It's hard. It's daunting. But then, once I start, it almost becomes a different sort of treasure hunt. Every mistake I find and correct is like a victory against some possible person in the future pouncing on me and calling my work sloppy.

I'd like to add one thing I do that might help other people writing nonfiction. Maybe everyone already does this and I'm the last to figure this out, but I keep a separate timeline for every section in my book. In it I list every fact and where I got it. I started doing this when I wrote the cold-case book because I was writing about so many different cases, with so many different "characters," detectives and other law enforcement personnel, and the cases I picked spanned a half century of time. So I had a hard time keeping track of what happened when, who did what, who said what, etc. These timelines helped me later when I had to go back and fact-check, but it wasn't the reason I started doing them. Now I am pretty meticulous about these timelines. I can't depend on them—the timelines are as vulnerable to error as anything else—but I at least know where to go back and check.

The Millions: Your first two books, *Cyberville* and *Waiting for My Cats to Die*, were definitely memoir. You followed those with *The Restless Sleep*, which is considered true crime, and your later books (*Unbelievable, Imperfect Harmony, Damnation Island*) seem to be more investigative and historical in nature. Can you talk about the arc of your nonfiction writing career, what made you turn from memoir to these other subjects? How is the writing process different for you in these very disparate non-fiction genres?

Stacy Horn: With the exception of *Cyberville*, all my books are different versions of the same quest or interests. But a quick backstory: I decided at nine years old that I wanted to be a writer, and originally I wanted to write novels. Fast-forward to the 1990s, when I started Echo, one of the early social networks, although we didn't call them that at the time. The *New York Times* did a brief profile of me, where I mentioned I wanted to be a writer and had an unpublished novel in my drawer. The next day I got a call from Warner Books, who said they'd publish my novel! Turns out, they didn't think it was publishable, but they liked my writing and they asked me if I wanted to write about the internet. My agent said do it. Once you have one book published it's easier to get another, and then you can try again to write a novel. That led to my first book, *Cyberville*, and the discovery that by writing nonfiction I could follow my interests and obsessions more directly than with fiction, and with much more satisfying results. And my biggest interests have to do with death and impermanence, and how many stories are forgotten. Every book circles back to this, at least to some extent, even if I begin by thinking they won't. Like my book about the history and joys of singing. Who knew that would be about death as well?

I pitched *Waiting for My Cats to Die* as a memoir, but it was always going to be about my first serious research into death and the fact that we and everyone and everything we love must die. *The Restless Sleep* was about people who not only had to die, they had their brief time on earth criminally cut short, and no one was answering for that. My book about the Parapsychology Laboratory of Duke University [*Unbelievable*] was supposed to be a fun break from death, but it turns out the lab was established in order to see if they could find evidence for life after death. My book about singing was also supposed to be a break, but our mortality is one of the driving inspirations for composers, musicians, and our audiences. We sing to deal with loss and to reaffirm life. Requiems are among the most moving and profound things I sing.

My books are my attempt to defy death and the fact that most of us will eventually be forgotten, and tragically quickly. It's a mission that will ultimately fail, but it's like singing requiems while I still can.

The Millions: I know this about your books, and about you, that often the theme (seems to be, anyway) is death. I'd like to draw your attention to some of your own quotes. From *Cyberville*: "As cyberspace grows, it will only become more and more like the rest of the world. Not an even bigger global village, but a bigger collection of villages." From *The Restless Sleep*: "I want to resurrect the city's forgotten dead." From *Imperfect Harmony*: "the magic current of potential that comes to life whenever people are drawn together by the astonishing and irresistible power of a song." Can I put it to you that your themes are actually community and resurrection and so much joy in life that even the hunt for its existence after it is gone is worthwhile?

Stacy Horn: Yes. Definitely. Community and resurrection. I'm not religious, so there is no hereafter for me (as far as I know). I think people who are religious think that makes life pointless and empty, and without the promise of heaven or the threat of hell there is no reason to be a good and decent person. But for me, the opposite is true. It makes life the only point, and therefore it's much more important to use it well, and to be as good a person as you can and not add misery and pain to anyone else's life. It's the only one they get.

Spending my time resurrecting forgotten lives, acknowledging past wrongs, feels meaningful to me. It does give me joy, and purpose to the now, and I hope it does the same for my readers. Knowing we're going to die, how do we want to live? What do we want to leave behind for the people who will replace us to use? What do we want to tell them? I want to tell them: "There was once this girl named Adelaide Irving. She was a lot like you."

Sarah Cords has only two interests: reading, and watching British TV. She blogs about the former at *Citizen Reader* and the latter at *The Great British TV Site*. This interview is published with the permission of Sarah Cords and *The Millions*.

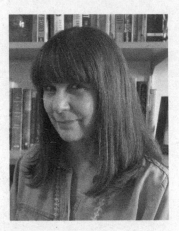

Stacy Horn is the author of five previous nonfiction books, including *Imperfect Harmony*. Mary Roach has hailed her for "combining awe-fueled curiosity with topflight reporting skills," while others have described her work as "immaculately researched" and "several notches above the typical reporter's insights."

Horn's commentaries have been heard on NPR's *All Things Considered*, and she is the founder of the social network Echo. She lives in New York City, and when she's not researching and writing, she's singing soprano 2 (the best part) with the Choral Society of Grace Church or helping care for animals at the ASPCA Animal Hospital, where she is frequently forced to chant quietly to herself, "No, Stacy, you may not take that puppy (or kitten) home." Her website is stacyhorn.com.